False Dawn

Critical Issues in Health and Medicine

Edited by Rima D. Apple, University of Wisconsin–Madison, and Janet Golden, Rutgers University–Camden

Growing criticism of the U.S. health-care system is coming from consumers, politicians, the media, activists, and health-care professionals. Critical Issues in Health and Medicine is a collection of books that explores these contemporary dilemmas from a variety of perspectives, among them political, legal, historical, sociological, and comparative, and with attention to crucial dimensions such as race, gender, ethnicity, sexuality, and culture.

For a list of titles in the series, see the last page of the book.

False Dawn

The Rise and Decline of Public Health Nursing

Karen Buhler-Wilkerson

Foreword by Susan M. Reverby and Julie A. Fairman

Rutgers University Press

New Brunswick, Camden, and Newark, New Jersey, and London

Library of Congress Cataloging-in-Publication Data

Name: Buhler-Wilkerson, Karen, 1944–2010, author.
Title: False dawn : the rise and decline of public health nursing / Karen Buhler-Wilkerson.
Description: New Brunswick : Rutgers University Press, [2021] | Series: Critical issues in health and medicine | Originally published: False dawn / Karen Buhler-Wilkerson. New York : Garland Pub., 1989. | Includes bibliographical references and index.
Identifiers: LCCN 2020012075 | ISBN 9781978808720 (paperback) | ISBN 9781978808737 (cloth) | ISBN 9781978808744 (epub) | ISBN 9781978808751 (mobi) | ISBN 9781978808768 (pdf)
Subjects: MESH: Public Health Nursing—history | History, 20th Century | United States
Classification: LCC RT97 | NLM WY 11 AA1 | DDC 610.73/4—dc23
LC record available at https://lccn.loc.gov/2020012075

A British Cataloging-in-Publication record for this book is available from the British Library.

False Dawn was first published by Garland Publishing, Inc. in 1989 as *False Dawn: The Rise and Decline of Public Health Nursing, 1900–1930*.

Copyright © 1989 by Karen Buhler-Wilkerson
Foreword copyright © 2021 by Susan M. Reverby and Julie A. Fairman
Suggested Readings copyright © 2021 by Sandra B. Lewenson
♾ The paper used in this publication meets the requirements of the American National Standard for Information Sciences—Permanence of Paper for Printed Library Materials, ANSI Z39.48-1992.

www.rutgersuniversitypress.org

Manufactured in the United States of America

For Ruth Buhler

Contents

Can There Be a New Dawn for Public Health Nursing?

The prominent issue in American health-care delivery in the early twentieth century became how to provide and control direct patient care to individuals and health promotion and disease prevention to populations.[1] As physicians became more organized and focused on the sanctity and economic control of the doctor-patient relationship, any intrusions from the state, voluntary associations, or other providers were viewed with alarm. The hospital as the site for acute, rather than chronic, care kept doctors lobbying to keep community-based health delivery at bay, where chronic ills might have better been addressed. As medical and public health education separated, these differences were exacerbated.[2]

Or so goes one of the standard historical articles on the divisions between medicine and public health.[3] Although this analysis is replete with photographs of nurses providing care, it leaves out their centrality to the tensions between institutional bedside care and community-based prevention and health promotion. And as we now continually attempt to understand why the United States spends more on health care yet has poorer rates of mortality and morbidity than other developed countries, we really need more of an analysis of the role nursing has played, or not played, in these developments. For public health, nurses may be a critical part of the solutions.[4]

Karen Buhler-Wilkerson's *False Dawn: The Rise and Decline of Public Health Nursing, 1900–1930*, first published in 1989 (Garland Press), filled the lacunae in this history for the first third of the twentieth century. Buhler-Wilkerson was prescient in understanding that the separation of health promotion and disease prevention from the care of those with both acute and chronic ills would fragment already divided delivery systems. She was able to analyze how nursing, too, was caught between its traditional role at the bedside and its expanding understanding that disease prevention and health promotion in the home and community were critical.

In the 1960s, sociologist Irving Zola disseminated the "stream" analogy for health care when he taught that we could not keep pulling drowning bodies out of a stream without focusing "upstream" to understand what made the bodies fall into the water.[5] Buhler-Wilkerson asked this question, without the stream metaphor, as she explored what happened to the promise of public health nursing and its ability to provide both individual care and community-based disease prevention and health promotion. In her analysis, the tensions among lay lady managers of the various voluntary associations who provided home care for the poor, the professionally trained nurse moving more into health education and prevention along with bedside care, the emphasis on fee-for-service payments, and the cutting of public funding all made the great promise of public health nursing impossible to fulfill.

Today, nursing education includes more exposure to clinical experiences and content on health education and prevention, although most nurses still work in hospitals, where their work remains siloed from the care nurses provide in the home and community. Accordingly, most of nursing education remains focused on acute care, although there are new community-based models slowly emerging. And nursing leaders' use of science as the way to gain legitimacy with hospitals, medical professionals, and frankly, patients still resonates in nursing curricula. Yet in the last decades, the science of public health has gained a great deal of traction with a new generation of nurses, policy makers, and health professional leaders who have "rediscovered" the importance of the upstream factors to the nation's health.

In *False Dawn*, Buhler-Wilkerson traced out the initial promise of public health nurses as they brought what they called "a message with their medicine." She examined the ways professionalizing nurses believed they could link scientific medicine and scientific charity through the work of the nurse outside of hospitals. Without using the term *social determinants of health* or *health disparities*, she explored how a determined group of nurses sought to make their middle-class-based public health teachings available to everyone across the class divide but ran up against the fee-for-service and charity models that made paying for such care difficult. As well, she noted how governments at the city and state levels failed to push for adequate funds to fulfill their responsibility to the public to protect their health or follow through by advancing protective legislation or implementing existing protective health and welfare laws.

Buhler-Wilkerson also traced out the divisions between the care provided by the voluntary groups of visiting nurse associations (VNAs; controlled by lady managers) and that provided by public health departments (controlled by public health physicians). Insurance companies weighed in as well, always searching for a cheaper nursing worker to visit their clients, while nurses fought to keep up their educational standards and become more efficient and effective in their practice.

By the 1920s, public health nurses, she argued, were up against the decline in infectious diseases, the legal limitations on immigration that shrank an important but not powerful constituency, and the growing importance of the hospital. Without a unified system that linked community care to hospitals, or a less fragmented and universal insurance program, alas public health nursing could do little to meet its promise or address the larger structural inequities and racism that undermined health unevenly throughout the American population.[6] Increasingly under the control of the public health doctors in official state agencies, the independence and promise of public health nursing started to fade. As Buhler-Wilkerson signaled with her title, the hope of a new day of linked patient care and population health-care promotion and prevention for nursing proved to be a "false dawn."

We lost this thoughtful historian, dedicated public health nurse, friend, and nursing professor to cancer in 2010, and so her intended follow-up for this book did not appear. She did produce an edited collection called *Nursing and the Public's Health: An Anthology of Sources* (1989). In her prize-winning, more focused monograph *No Place like Home: A History of Nursing and Home Care in the United States* (2001), she returned to these queries. Here, she chronicled the fragmentation and refusal to provide (as well as pay for) proper home care for those with both acute and chronic illnesses. This volume also focused more on the racism inherent in the ways this country has organized its fragmented health-care system.[7]

In the decade since Buhler-Wilkerson's passing, there is still no comprehensive book on the relationships among medicine, public health nursing, and the fall and rise of public health. Had Buhler-Wilkerson been able to write a second volume, we suspect she would have looked more closely at the failures of public health expansion during the Great Depression, the piecemeal funding for care for women and children, health care in schools, occupational health and safety, and rural health care. She probably would have addressed the huge Hill-Burton funding of hospitals in the post–World War II era, combined with the

expansion of research at the National Institutes of Health, or the link between
the Centers for Disease Control and Prevention (CDC) and the rise of big pharma,
which caused home care and public health to yet again take a back seat.[8]

Part of the post–World War II loss of the public health safety net came from
the public enthusiasm whipped up by media and advertising for new drugs,
treatments, and modern hospitals, as well as a new type of individualism that
was wrapped up in consumerism.[9] Health was something to be purchased. As
more people gained private hospital insurance through their workplace—an
outcome of the Supreme Court decision in *Inland Steel v. The National Labor
Relations Board* case in 1948 and postwar wage controls—they also claimed
their rights to the best and most advanced care.[10] Public health nursing survived in places where these changes were not felt or experienced—poor rural
communities and impoverished urban areas. Black public health nurses were
sometimes the only health-care providers available to black rural southern and
northern urban communities.[11]

Efforts to refocus on community-based care and public health in the 1960s
came with additional funding through the auspices of federal agencies such as
the Office of Economic Opportunity, the Public Health Service, or the Department of Housing and Urban Development.[12] Community-based care and public
participation also became a critical part of a political and altruistic struggle for
health-care rights in the 1970s against the "welfare colonialism" of the 1960s.[13]
Although funding for public health through community projects increased, as
seen by the rise of community health centers and the funding of community
health and home health aides, it led to, as critics noted, "tiny band aids for
everyone or continuity of care for a few."[14]

Many community-based models of care emerged during the 1970s, and
many times physicians were credited with this movement. Public health
nurses were crucial activists, although often ignored by many of the histories.[15] Even so, public health nurses still carried a "message with their medicine," and many joined the social movements of the 1960s and 1970s to fight
for social justice.

Activist groups and political movements from the Catholic Alexian Brothers, the Black Panthers, Latinx groups in the Southwest, and the more urban-
based Young Lords in New York and Chicago captured the opportunities the
turmoil of these decades offered to activists of all persuasions.[16] Although such
political groups focused attention on what our fragmented health system was
not accomplishing, most of the clinics they created were fleeting as funds dried
up in the late 1960s and early 1970s. By the 1970s, the inflation of the Vietnam
War years and the oil boycott caught up with the American economy. What was

labeled as the "fiscal crisis of the state" devastated much of public health funding and infrastructure at the state level.[17]

The feminist health clinics of the 1970s also renewed the focus on public
health through the targeting of medical paternalism and overall dissatisfaction
with physician providers. Many women wanted more and better information to
make their own decisions about their health, broadly construed as birth control, medication side effects, and in the most basic terms, information about
their own bodies. Public health nurses, including nurse midwives, were seen
as frontline experts along with feminist lay health advocates, although nurses
in acute care institutions in general were not given this acknowledgment. The
feminist health movement also provided many women an entry into nursing
through nurse practitioner programs and baccalaureate programs for those with
undergraduate degrees in other fields, which gave them the skills to practice
their feminist ideals in communities of women.

Just as the cities and states were pulling out of the austerity in the 1980s,
the HIV/AIDS crisis hit. Homophobia, sexism, and racism hardly prepared an
underfunded public health sector to deal with its biggest infectious disease
problem since the epidemics of influenza (1918) and polio (1950s). This time,
however—perhaps because of the gay population it affected at first as well as
the fears that normative heterosexuals might be the next victims—public health
nursing went into the breach created by fear. Public health nurses—gay, les-
bian, trans, and straight—were some of the earliest caretakers of victims as well
as critical data gatherers to determine the causes and strategies for prevention
during the epidemic. These nurses have also been part of the efforts to provide appropriate prevention and care as the HIV/AIDS epidemic has become a
global pandemic.[18]

Other epidemics, such as drug abuse, gun violence, high infant and maternal mortality rates associated with the stress of prolonged exposure to racism,
and the growth of chronic diseases in the last decades, have shaken our faith
in the ability of our acute care–focused health system to improve health. A
well-resourced and capable public health system with a well-educated workforce of public health nurses is needed to collect data, inform and educate the
public, identify and solve health issues, and target populations that may benefit from early intervention strategies. Although health promotion and disease
prevention are the cornerstones of public health, these issues are also tightly
connected to the provision of individual care. Public health nurses could help
bridge this age-old divide.[19]

We need to recall that an acute care system does not focus "upstream."
As we have seen in the Flint, Michigan, water crises, public health scientists,

nurses, and teachers, rather than acute care institutions, raised public aware-
ness of the need for a strong public health system and an adequate workforce
of public health nurses to anticipate and identify problems related to particular
communities/populations.[20]

Public health issues are also being redefined: the explosion of police violence against black men, women, and children and their out-of-proportion
incarceration are now defined as public health issues.[21] While more recently
public health officials have called mass incarceration, lack of housing, and racism "public health problems," we do not yet have much of a history of this
from the nursing perspective. Furthermore, we are just beginning to have more
information on the impact of the climate crisis on human health as we face heat
waves, more turbulent weather, and lack of water across the globe.[22]

Many of these problems are embedded in the effects of upstream factors
that public health nurses identified so many years ago. Even so, we have seen
a startling but much needed renewed focus on these factors, as seen in semi-
nal reports from the National Academy of Medicine,[23] the U.S. Department of
Health and Human Services,[24] and the CDC.[25] The terrible COVID-19 pandemic
of 2020 has exposed these limitations of the much-vaunted American health-
care system even more. The lack of support for testing, contact tracing, and
health education has made nurses into martyrs in our hospitals as the structural
factors that exacerbate who gets sick and who dies are still so unaddressed.

Although many see this focus on upstream factors as something new, innovative, and unique, Buhler-Wilkerson's work remains timely in reminding us
we have been here before. The public health nurses she wrote about recognized
and tried to manage some of the same problems in the populations they cared
for and in the neighborhoods they monitored. Adequate resources, clean water,
safe neighborhoods, and access to nutritious foods, as well as expert care, are
historic continuities for those nurses who tried to better the lives of immigrant
urban and rural communities in the early decades of the twentieth century.[26]

As historians Theodore Brown and Elizabeth Fee have argued, social movements in health have been crucial to improvements in public health, not merely
"biomedical advances and administrative improvements."[27] The connections
between public health nurses and health activists need more historical consideration. It has become clearer that without the links between providers and
activists, very little changes in health policy.[28] The current debate over "Medicare for All," for example, would never have happened without the agitation
for differing kinds of payment schemes that has gone on for years, some of
which has been spearheaded by nurses.[29] The growing recognition that we now
face the twin pandemics of racism and COVID-19 perhaps will help change the

focus to the upstream factors that make people sick and for which there is no medical cure.

With the renewed focus on public health, we have the opportunity to maximize the potential of public health nurses. Whereas fragmentation of work in the early decades of the twentieth century prevented a cohesive and organized strategy to address public health, better organized and integrated systems of both public and private funding and payment for services could create the foundation for a more seamless system. For example, the Philadelphia Visiting Nurses Association, one of Buhler-Wilkerson's cases, has a renewed focus now on population-based care with its ability to provide nutritious food deliveries by nurses through its relationship with food pantries and data systems that help identify population-based health issues in communities into which few other organizations want to venture because of the low reimbursement rates and overwhelming social problems. The agency works closely with acute care institutions toward a common goal of keeping people out of the hospital and as healthy as possible.

Public health nurses, as part of not-for-profit (and for-profit alike) home care agencies, except for the nurses who work at the CDC, rarely find their employment with government agencies today. They work for home health agencies, hospitals, and sometimes state agencies. And in a reversal of the trend in the first decades of the twentieth century because of recent Medicare regulations, more care is moving into the home as acute care institutions are now penalized for patient readmissions within thirty days of their original discharge. Public health nurses are seeing their experiences and their principles more highly valued than in earlier decades as they and other types of nurses are sought out to help institutions operationalize the new regulations.

Public health nurses are needed to strengthen the connection between a patient's experience in the hospital and his health habits at home or in his community, even as more patients are discharged from hospital care needing much nursing attention. Buhler-Wilkerson showed how the movement of patients into hospital care as well as the conflicts between public and private organizations over the control of the work of public health nurses doomed what could have been the "dawn" of public health nursing. The movement of patients out of hospitals or prevention of their admission through population-based care in the home or community reverses this historic factor: it could offer a new dawn of public health nursing.

Such nurses have the skills and knowledge to work in teams and to develop individual and community-based plans for combatting some of the most pervasive (and continuous) health problems we face as a society, as well as serving as a model for how to bridge the divide between individual and population-based care. In a recent discussion with public health nurses, we found they still identify some of the same issues Buhler-Wilkerson noted in the early decades of the twentieth century: lacking adequate resources, seeing themselves as the safety net for marginalized populations—the last and first line of defense—and grappling with the health and ethical issues of our approaches to the homeless, migrants, and immigrants. The nurses understand the weaknesses and gaps they see every day in our fragmented system as they try to provide care to the public in their homes and communities, and they are still a group of nurses who fight for social justice for their patients. The work they do provides the foundation for a healthier public even in the absence of adequate resources, and they are quite good at creating a pathway to health with few resources.[30]

We end as Buhler-Wilkerson closed her own preface: this work is still a critical resource for those who are "struggling to design a more viable public health system."[31] As Buhler-Wilkerson posited, public health nurses may be our best answer to coalesce our fragmented health system, but they will need the support of nursing education, policy makers, insurers, and healthcare institutions to fulfill their promise. And as early twentieth-century and modern public health nurses understand, the struggle for social justice should be a critical thread of their work and their message. They cannot, however, do it alone; they need to be united with others pushing for equality and justice in health care. The question remains, How can nurses accomplish this, and who will provide the necessary resources?

Susan M. Reverby
Julie A. Fairman

Preface

Confronted by the AIDS epidemic, an unacceptable level of infant mortality, the unmet needs of the medically indigent, a growing number of elderly afflicted by chronic, degenerative diseases, and the rising costs of health care, contemporary health analysts have begun to wonder where and how to respond to these new patterns of need and morbidity. One of the most recent reactions to this set of concerns is the Institute of Medicine's study *The Future of Public Health*. Defining the mission of public health as "fulfilling society's interest in assuring conditions in which people can be healthy," the authors conclude that our current public health system is in disarray.[1]

Most analysts, unaware of the circumstances that have shaped this field's history, ironically fail to realize that many of our contemporary complexities are not new. Both the current lack of consensus as to the mission of public health and the inability of many communities to take effective public health action suggest that we are revisiting earlier unsolved dilemmas. The solutions we seek will no doubt be shaped by the legacies of these earlier experiences.

Although, in recent years, much has been learned about the history of public health, few historians considered nursing's contributions to this past—whether good or bad.[2] The aim of this study is to provide a historical analysis of the origins and subsequent development of public health nursing in the United States between the 1880s and the Depression of the 1930s.

Public health nursing began in small, local undertakings in which a few wealthy women hired one or two nurses to visit the sick poor in their homes. The nurses aimed to care for the sick, teach the family how to care for the patient, and above all, protect the public from the spread of disease through forceful, yet tactful, lessons in healthful living. The ailments they encountered were frequently infectious, often acute, and always complicated by the social and economic circumstances of the family. By 1910, the work of these nurses expanded to include a variety of preventive programs for schoolchildren, infants, mothers, and patients with tuberculosis. Acting as a self-conscious "missionary of health," the public health nurse tried to translate the knowledge of scientific medicine into concepts of disease prevention and personal responsibility for health.

Although most preventive programs were originated by voluntary organizations, such as visiting nurse associations (VNAs), they were eventually taken over by public boards of health and education. The development of preventive services varied from city to city; voluntary and governmental agencies were unpredictable and often overlapping in their shared health-care responsibilities. As the confusion grew, so did the debate concerning the appropriate functions of voluntary versus governmental health agencies.

The struggle between voluntary and public organizations was not the only dispute hampering public health practice. Attempts by health departments to extend their health care focus resulted in conflict with the medical profession as well. Inevitably, most health departments were forced to abandon claims to any curative activities construed as threatening the economic well-being of private physicians. Consequently, despite much ongoing discussion, health departments and school health services became increasingly preventive in scope. An inescapable, though seemingly unexpected, consequence of this development was the limitation of publicly funded nurses' activities to the prevention of disease, while the care of the sick was left to the voluntary agencies, especially the VNAs.

Developing under the aegis of both publicly funded and voluntary organizations, public health nursing was too fragmented to generate an institutional framework that allowed these nurses to care for both the healthy and the sick. Although the nursing leadership campaigned for the creation of comprehensive, coordinated, community-based nursing services, little changed. Despite the failure of their ideal, public health nurses went on caring for at least some of the public—in sickness or in health but rarely the same nurse for both.

By the late 1920s, public health nursing reached a turning point. From the perspective of the VNAs, the circumstances that had created a need for their organizations a mere two decades before were simply no longer of major concern to most communities. Urban death rates continued to decline, and infectious diseases were being replaced by chronic, degenerative diseases as leading causes of death. Chronic diseases did not appear in epidemic form, creating the kind of fluctuating and often frightening impact that originally prompted public concern and philanthropic support for these nurses. Simultaneously, medical, surgical, and even some obstetrical patients of all social classes began to seek hospital-based care. The growing centrality of the hospital meant that fewer patients sick at home would require the services of a trained nurse. As their original purpose and mission became increasingly elusive, support for these visiting nurses began to peak.

Throughout this period, nursing in governmental agencies continued to expand. By 1924, with 54 percent of all public health nurses working in governmental health agencies, it seemed inevitable that governmental organizations would become the major source of employment for the field. In publicly funded jobs, the nurses found support for their traditional concerns—infectious diseases and health education for the poor. Yet as medical and public interest shifted away from these problems, public health nurses could not hold the central place within the health-care system that had once, albeit briefly, been theirs.

This historical study critically analyzes why a movement that might have become a significant vehicle for delivering comprehensive health care to the American public failed to reach its potential. Chapter 1 is a brief examination of the origins of public health nursing, first in England and later in the United States. Although little information exists about these nurses or their patients, in this chapter, I try to provide a sketch of both. What results is primarily a description of the nurses' work and their attitudes toward their largely immigrant clients.

Chapter 2 examines the changing relationships between the ladies who organized, funded, and managed these organizations and the nurses they hired. Chapter 3 explores the effect of the "new public health movement" on nursing. Here the creation of this new nursing role as well as the specialization and the separation of bedside care of the sick from the teaching of prevention that followed are considered.

Chapter 4 looks at the origins of the National Organization for Public Health Nursing (NOPHN) and the American Red Cross Rural Nursing Service. The effect of World War I upon both of these organizations and VNAs is also discussed in this chapter. The final chapter analyzes the decline of public health nursing during the late 1920s.

Throughout these chapters, I have relied on the records of the NOPHN and the Public Health Nursing Section of the American Public Health Association (APHA), the papers and writings of the public health nursing leadership, major studies of public health nursing, numerous unpublished reports, the records of the Welfare Division of the Metropolitan Life Insurance Company (MLI), and a careful reading of the major nursing and public health journals during this period. For a more accurate understanding of local institutions and issues, I have depended heavily upon the records of the VNAs of Philadelphia, Boston, Providence, and to a lesser extent, those of the Cleveland and New York agencies.

Because public health nursing developed within both voluntary organizations, where the primary concern was the care of the sick at home, and public agencies, where nurses served as ambassadors of health education to the poor, the field provides a still unexplored view of the practice of medicine, nursing, and public health prior to the Depression. More precisely, this history of public health nursing can be interpreted as a case study of the transformation of the care of the sick from the home to the hospital, the changing emphasis of the field of public health from sanitation to preventive programs, and the conflicts that developed between public and voluntary health agencies as they struggled to develop cooperative relationships within their shared domains.

While earlier histories of nursing have tended to emphasize praise and the recounting of progress, this study examines both victories and defeats. But in so doing, my intent has been, to borrow the words of Shirley Anne Williams, more to examine the character and consciousness of these nurses and their organizations than to learn who trampled on them—for we already know too well the how and why of that reality. Rather, as Williams has suggested, my concern has been "to learn what our mothers planted there, what they thought as they sowed, and how they survived the blighting of so many fruits."[3]

My ability to achieve this task has been greatly enhanced by the recent work of several historians of medicine and nursing. In particular, Susan Reverby's study of nursing has provided invaluable direction to my own inquiry, often causing me to ask questions I would have otherwise ignored. Although I did not always arrive at the same conclusions, I found Barbara Melosh's analysis of public health nursing most useful. Likewise, the work of Charles Rosenberg, Janet Wilson James, Nancy Tomes, and Susan Armeny provided a great deal of clarity to particular issues I would have otherwise not understood. I hope, in turn, that this study will be helpful both to those interested in acquiring a more complete understanding of the past and to those struggling to design a more viable public health system.

False Dawn

Chapter 1

Trained Nurses for the Sick Poor

Care, Cleanliness, and Character

By the end of the nineteenth century, a "new power for good" had been added to the armament of those fighting the moral and social disintegration brought on, they contended, by industrialization, urbanization, and immigration. Motivated by a shared "vision" of the good society, wealthy ladies in New York, Philadelphia, Boston, Buffalo, and Chicago hired trained nurses to visit the homes of the sick poor. At first, they were unaware of their parallel activities, for these ladies modeled their new charity organizations after the English idea of district nursing.[1]

In the English system, cities were divided into manageable districts, each with its own nurse whose work was supervised and financed by wealthy and concerned local citizens. The benefits of these nurses' visits were found to go far beyond simply relieving the pain and misery of sickness, for in treating the illness of one family member, nurses were given an opportunity to reform and re-create the whole family. Thus the district nurse seemed an appealing solution to the complex problem of elevating poor families to a more ordered and healthier realm of moral and physical well-being.

Not surprisingly, the idea of the district nurse appealed both to American philanthropists seeking to restore order to the city as well as to a newly emerging nursing leadership striving for recognition as a profession. Even though by the 1890s only thirty-five associations had been established in this country, support was rapidly growing and the future seemed to hold great promise for this new field.

While the image of the visiting nurse climbing the tenement stairs to save the indigent from illness and bad habits struck the fancy of many social

reformers, the demands of the actual work often proved extreme. The combination of crowded tenements, language problems, "foreign" ideas, acute illness,
and exposure to inclement weather simply did not appeal to all nurses. As a
result, the turnover in many visiting nurse associations (VNAs) was high. But
for those nurses who endured, the work proved both challenging and reward-
ing. This chapter briefly examines the evolution of district nursing in England
and the United States, its relationship to the needs of many turn-of-the-century
urban industrial communities, and the nature of the work undertaken by these
nurses.

I

By the last decades of the nineteenth century, many American cities were expe-
riencing a major transformation. Those first affected were the northern coastal
cities where the concentration of immigrants and industry made poverty, disease, and dirt unavoidable. Population growth alone required major adjust-
ments in the lives of most of these city dwellers, even those able to escape to
newer, less crowded neighborhoods.

    With immigration accounting for much of this urban growth, ethnic, cul-
tural, religious, and economic differences accentuated the separation between
old and new inhabitants. For many, the shattered patterns of a once cohesive
city life and the growing distance between the classes that resulted caused
apprehension. From the perspective of the wealthy, immigrants were perceived
as a profound threat to the social and moral order.[2] In their search for solutions
to these urban threats, a variety of strategies were implemented to stave off
moral, social, and physical disintegration among the urban masses.[3] Out of a
fundamentally similar set of convictions about the cause and cure of poverty
would evolve scores of charitable organizations—among them the idea of the
visiting nurse.

    One of the significant motivating forces during this period was a belief that
the roots of urban poverty lay in the moral deficiencies and character flaws
of the poor. With the circumstances of city life having cut them off from the
elevating influence of their moral betters, the argument followed that the poor
had been left without the means to recognize and correct their deficiencies.
Irresistibly drawn by these ideas, thousands of upper- and middle-class ladies
volunteered to expand the moral conduit between the classes by visiting a
small number of carefully selected slum families. The key to urban America's
moral redemptions had, at last, been found in the support of "true friendship."[4]

    Unfortunately, the friendly visitor armed with the tenets of scientific char-
ity found herself defenseless when confronted with disease. Despite declining

death rates, late nineteenth-century American cities were unhealthy places to live. In most, seventeen out of every one thousand persons died each year, fifteen out of every one hundred infants never lived to reach one year of age, and the average life expectancy was only a bit more than forty years. City dwellers found themselves living with the ever-present threats of influenza, pneumonia, typhus, typhoid fever, summer fever, smallpox, scarlet fever, measles, whooping cough, dysentery, and tuberculosis. The greatest killer among them was tuberculosis.[5]

For those ladies who realized, with the advent of the germ theory of disease, that their health depended to some extent at least on the health of the rest of the population, the hazard of infectious diseases must have seemed a much more tangible concern than any defect in the character or ambitions of the poor. The knowledge that the diseases of workers who sewed clothes in their filthy tenement homes or who processed food could spread to decent, clean, and respectable citizens served as a powerful incentive for renewed efforts to eliminate the menace of illness among the poor, particularly the immigrants.[6]

While the diseases of the middle and upper classes were supervised by the frequent visits of the family physician either in their homes or, to a lesser extent, in the well-ordered surroundings of a hospital's pay ward or private rooms, the activities of the poor during illness seemed by comparison carelessly regulated. Eager to avoid hospitalization, the urban poor often chose to stay at home during illnesses, relying on traditional healing methods or, perhaps, the services of the dispensary physician.[7]

For a few lady philanthropists (Mrs. William Osburn of New York, Abbie Howes and Phoebe Adams of Boston, Mrs. William Furness Jenks of Philadelphia, Elizabeth Marshall of Buffalo, and Clarissa Shumway of Chicago), this system of care that left the poor to struggle with illness as best they could in their crowded and dirty tenement homes was intolerable.[8] Following the English example, they looked to the trained nurse to bring care, cleanliness, and character to the homes of the sick poor. For, as was the case with so many philanthropic activities, visiting nurses were expected to bring a message with their medicine. Disciplined and well-bred women, they were to raise the "household existence" with their "delicate instruction and firm convictions" and to protect the public from the spread of disease with forceful yet tactful lessons in physical and moral hygiene. In the visiting nurse had at last been found "the safest and most practical means of bridging the gulf which lies between the classes and the masses."[9]

II

The English model, which so enamored the American lady philanthropists, had been created as a seemingly logical extension of the friendly visitor's efforts to check "the rising tide of pauperism." The first attempt to send trained nurses into the homes of the sick poor was initiated in Liverpool in 1859 under the direction of William Rathbone, a wealthy Quaker philanthropist and businessman.[10]

Rathbone was first exposed to the phenomenon of the trained nurse during the long and painful illness of his wife. Amazed by the degree of comfort and ease of suffering provided by a nurse's care in the most luxurious of circumstances, he wondered what even greater degree of alleviation she might produce in the less comfortable homes of the poor. Eager to try out this idea, he convinced Mary Robinson, his wife's nurse, to participate in just such an experiment. Consistent with Rathbone's views of constructive charitable intervention, Robinson was instructed to care for the sick while simultaneously teaching them how to better care for themselves.[11]

Shocked and overwhelmed by the hopeless misery and poverty she encountered, Robinson tried, reportedly, to terminate the experiment before the end of their three-month agreement. Encouraged by her employer to continue, she eventually agreed, and in the end, they both declared the project a great success. In the words of Rathbone, the hopeless were restored to health and breadwinners and mothers to independence, while the spread of weakness and disease were halted. Nursing had, he exclaimed, demonstrated its ability to prevent the "moral ruin, the recklessness, the drunkenness and the crime which so often follow upon hopeless misery."[12]

Having experienced such a successful beginning, Rathbone saw it as his duty to extend the benefits of the trained nurse to all Liverpool's poor. Unfortunately, his ability to create support for his new enterprise far exceeded the available supply of trained nurses. By 1861, he turned in desperation to Florence Nightingale.[13]

Nightingale saw the care of the sick poor in their homes as one of nursing's most important tasks and willingly lent her support to his new enterprise. What followed was a voluminous correspondence between the two. Nightingale gave Rathbone's plans her close and constant consideration, publishing her earliest ideas on the subject in his 1865 *Organization of Nursing in a Large Town*. But it was her 1874 paper "Suggestions for Improving the Nursing Service of Hospitals and on the Method of Training Nurses for the Sick Poor" that promoters of the field most often turned to for guidance.[14]

Two years later, her widely read letter to the *Times* "Untrained Nursing for the Sick Poor" made the district nurses' work for the first time well-known to the public. In this, her plea for their financial support, she told of the "depauperizing" effect of the trained nurse on the lives of the sick poor. These new visitors to the homes of the poor were not, she assured her readers, some new form of cooks, relief officers, district visitors, letter writers, general storekeepers, upholsterers, almoners, purveyors, ladies bountiful, head dispensers, or medical comforts shops; they were simply nurses. These nurses would achieve laudable results, she claimed, first by nursing and second by scouring dens of foulness, dirt, and vermin into the tidy, airy rooms required for recovery. When other forms of relief were required, the nurse knew how and where to apply for them, but her real task was simple and straightforward: "To set these poor sick people going again," suggested Nightingale, "with a sound and clean house, as well as with a sound body and mind, is about as great a benefit as we can give them—worth acres of gifts and relief."[15]

While willingly offering Rathbone advice and direction, Nightingale could find him no trained nurses. The only solution, she concluded, was for Rathbone to form his own school of nursing. His efforts proved successful, and only four years after their initiation, trained nurses were available throughout Liverpool. Rathbone organized his nursing service in the same fashion he approached the giving of relief: on a district basis under the supervision of ladies. Thus nursing of the sick poor in their homes came to be known as district nursing. As in other forms of relief giving, the presence of ladies guaranteed that the work of the nurses would be supported by appropriate patient records, financial accounts, and most importantly, money.[16]

Thanks to the success of the district nurse in Liverpool, nursing of the sick poor grew in popularity throughout England. But to the alarm of some, it gradually became an activity that both trained and untrained nurses were hired to pursue. By 1874, a committee, chaired by Rathbone, had been appointed to consider the question of providing more fully trained nurses for this work. At the suggestions of Nightingale, Florence Lee, one of the first pupils of the Nightingale school, was selected to conduct the investigation. The year-long study that resulted was financed by Rathbone and proved to be the first of many such inquiries.[17]

Lee, like her mentor Nightingale, went in search of facts and statistics. She wanted to know what district nurses did, their training for this work, and the quality and amount of service they provided. What she found was that the nurses were taken from "the lower grade of women" and that their work generally lacked "regulation" and, as a result, was often open to "grave objections."

Host nurses with whom she visited were not, in her estimation, well enough trained to be trusted to care for the sick in their homes. They tended to lapse into slovenliness and neglect, nursing too little while giving too much relief; they communicated too little with doctors and not infrequently acted, in the absence of medical supervision, more like doctors than nurses. Finally, they failed to instruct the patient's family and friends in the care of the sick or the necessary preventive and sanitary measures.[18]

She found the responsibilities of the district nurse were simply much greater than those of the carefully supervised private-duty nurse with a doctor close at hand and all the "appliances" necessary for the patients' care. While an additional three to six months' training in district work seemed an immediate solution, she concluded that, in the future, district nurses would need both to receive more education and to come from a higher "grade of women." Reforming and re-creating the homes of the poor were simply too difficult for nurses who came from the same class as their patients. Gentlewomen, she concluded, were most suited for this work since they could call upon the influence provided by their higher social position and likewise would be most content to be "servants of the sick poor" and "teacher[s] by turns." Reciprocally, of all employments open to gentlewomen, none, submitted Lee, were more suitable than district nursing.[19]

Lee's final recommendation was that district nurses be provided with a common home, one that supported them morally, materially, and spiritually, for no woman should be expected to come home "dog tired" from her patients and have to cook and clean. To create a home for the poor, she argued, the nurse must have a fit home for herself. Otherwise, it was like asking women who had forgotten what a home was to reconstruct the homes of the poor. Finally, the head of these homes would be a nurse "pre-eminently trained and skilled" who would provide the nurses with training, supervision, support, and sympathy in their common work. In short, what would result was a home for nurses where any good mother, of whatever class, would be willing to let her daughter, however attractive or highly educated, live.[20]

The report, published June 11, 1875, was widely read and in such demand that it was soon reprinted. While the committee and Nightingale wholeheartedly supported most of Lee's conclusions, they viewed her endorsement of the gentlewoman as a savior of district nursing with some skepticism. They agreed, nevertheless, to give her methods a try for a "year or so." Lee was asked to implement her plans as superintendent general of the Metropolitan and National Nursing Association for Providing Trained Nurses for the Sick Poor,

which was created the following winter in London. Ultimately, the committee claimed that their decision to support Lee's recommendations was proven
correct.[21]

Even though Lee resigned from this position in 1879 when she married
the Reverend Dacre Craven, she and her husband's efforts on behalf of district
nursing continued to shape the field's development. By 1889, what she had
established in England remained the standard emulated by American nursing
leaders for the next three decades.[22]

Finally, through the Cravens' efforts, the Queen's Jubilee Committee agreed
to use funds raised in celebration of Queen Victoria's fifty-year reign for the
training and support of district nursing throughout the country. Having gained
Victoria's approval of their efforts, seven thousand pounds of the fund were
designated for this purpose. In September 1889, after many months of prelimi-
nary labor, the Queen Victoria Jubilee Institute for Nurses was established by
royal charter, and district nursing associations throughout the British Isles were
invited to affiliate. All the principle organizations readily accepted. Through
the creation of what one author called "one grand system," all the unrelated
work that had developed throughout the country was brought under the control of this standardized national organization. In exchange for conforming to
uniform standards of "efficiency and training," affiliated associations received
help, advice, temporary financial aid, and regular supervision by a trained
nurse inspector. They were also supplied with a fully trained district nurse
as rapidly as the institute could turn them out. At Craven's suggestion, these
nurses were known as the "Queen's Nurses."[23]

III

Guided by English precedent, the introduction of district nursing in this country was, moreover, a logical extension of church-based urban philanthropy that
had dominated the preceding generation.[24] Although the convictions of religious benevolent organizations were being replaced by those of the nonsec-
tarian charity organization, settlement houses and dispensary movements, all
recognized the value of working in the actual homes of the poor. Thus district
nursing was a consistent development that followed in the American tradition
of friendly visiting.[25]

Not surprisingly, the first trained nurse to enter the homes of the sick poor
was a "missionary nurse" sent in 1877 by the women's branch of the New York
Mission and Tract Society. While the aim of this first visiting nurse was to
seek every opportunity to "elevate" her patients, morally and physically, the

primary intent of her work was to "lead souls to Christ." A few months later, similar work was initiated by New York's United Relief Works Society for Ethical Culture whose nurses worked under the direction of the New York Dispensary's physicians.[26]

By the 1880s, America had, as one early visiting nurse recalled, "caught the reflection of England's light." In fact, two of the oldest and most influential organizations, in Boston and Philadelphia, were actually created as a direct response to accounts of the success of district nursing in England.[27]

The Boston association, the Instructive District Nursing Association (IDNA), was founded by two friends, Howe and Adams, as a cooperative arrangement with the Boston Dispensary. The plan to introduce district nursing in Boston originated in 1884 with Howe, who had for years been a friendly visitor for Boston's Associated Charities. Learning of the work in England, she convinced Adams, the Women's Education Association, and eventually the Boston Dispensary to support this new undertaking. Eager to learn more of the English system of district nursing, Howe and Adams initiated what would become an active correspondence with Rathbone.[28]

By February 8, 1886, the ladies had opened their first office in "a spare corner" in the dispensary and had hired their first nurse, Miss Amelia Hodgkiss. The number of patients grew so rapidly that by April, a second nurse, Miss C. E. M. Somerville, was employed, and by November, a third nurse had been added to the staff. Each nurse's work was directed by her district's dispensary physician, with whom she met each morning to plan the day's work. This arrangement proved most successful, and by the end of the year, 7,182 visits had been made to 707 patients. After two years, the association was incorporated with a governing board of fifteen lady managers.[29]

The same month the Boston ladies were sending out their first nurse, Jenks of Philadelphia found herself being entertained during a "long stormy day in February, 1886" by a houseguest's report of her work with the district nurses in Manchester, England. This was, so the story goes, an entirely new idea for which Jenks felt a great deal of enthusiasm. Assured by her English friend that, if properly organized, this work would produce much good among the poor while only requiring a morning or possibly one day a week of a few ladies' time, Jenks decided such an undertaking sounded well worth the effort. By the following month, she had brought together a board of directors and a trained nurse.[30]

Unlike the Boston association, the ladies in Philadelphia spent much of their first year searching for both patients and funds. Despite the encouragement of a few physicians, such as James Hutchison and S. Weir Mitchell, they received little support from the city's charity organizations, physicians, or even their "philanthropic friends" for the idea of the visiting nurse. By the end of the first year, their nurse had only cared for 380 patients.[31]

While in several large cities ladies were quietly beginning similar endeavors, Isabel Hampton had taken for herself the task of becoming the nursing profession's earliest public champion of the district nurse. Hampton, it seems, was uniquely qualified, by both opportunity and ability, for this mission. She had first heard of this new nursing practice field while still in Chicago during her last year as the superintendent of nurses at the Illinois Training School. Shortly thereafter, she moved to Baltimore, having won the coveted post as first superintendent of the prestigious Johns Hopkins Hospital Training School for Nurses.[32]

Even in her new and demanding position, Hampton retained her interest in district nursing, encouraged no doubt by such like-minded members of the Hopkins medical staff as William Welch. Like Hampton, Welch saw medical care for the poor as not only altruistic but a wise investment for any community. He even had visions of a major institute of hygiene at Hopkins.[33]

Hampton's views on district nursing apparently began to crystallize after her visit to Boston's IDNA during the spring of 1890. Here, under the "kindly escort" of one of the lady managers, she claimed she was able to obtain a broader understanding of the work of the district nurses and "considerable insight into their methods." Hampton recognized in this new kind of work for nurses the potential for both fulfilling the womanly mission of social uplift and the promise of enhancing the status of nursing. Hampton realized that district nursing was the one field where nursing could, on its own, attain a distinct social importance; unlike their hospital-based sisters, these nurses working alone in the homes of the poor occupied center stage. It was, according to Hampton, the "highest type of nursing."[34]

In her new position, Hampton found numerous opportunities to share her concepts of nursing with the public, and not surprisingly, the importance of the district nurse was a recurring theme. For example, in May 1890, when she became the first nurse to address the influential National Conference of Charities and Corrections, her paper emphasized the nurse's role in both scientific medicine and the contemporary vision of scientific charity.[35]

That summer, while on vacation in England, she observed the English system during a visit to the central home and training school for district nurses in North London. The next year, in a talk to the Baltimore Charity Organization Society, she told her audience of her travels. Sharing her views on district nursing and her assessment of the importance of the work she had observed, she urged their support for the introduction of this new branch of philanthropy in Baltimore.[36]

The meeting of the International Congress of Charities, Correction and Philanthropy, which met in Chicago at the 1893 World's Fair, presented Hampton with her next opportunity to shape her profession's future. Hopkins-affiliated physicians dominated the congress's special sessions on hospitals, with John Shaw Billings serving as chairman, and when it was decided to have a nursing session, Billings offered the chair to Hampton.[37]

Lavinia Dock, her assistant at Hopkins, would later recount how Hampton through "most earnest thought and divination" went through the process of "construction of the entire subsequent evolution of the nursing profession." As a result, in the program could be found "the seedlings of almost all the later lines of growth" in the profession in the United States. According to Dock, "She placed the papers so that certain ideas should be worked out, and waited almost breathlessly for the results she hoped for."[38]

The array of papers and presenters was indeed impressive, and while district nursing did not dominate the session, it received ample attention. Three of the four speakers on district nurses were English, presumably a reflection of English prestige and experience. The English speakers were Nightingale (in absentia), Amy Hughes, and Mrs. Dacre Craven (Florence Lee). The fourth paper on district nurses in the United States was presented by Somerville, the second nurse to work for the IDNA of Boston. Consistent with Hampton's views, all the speakers stressed the important role of the district nurse, the need for district nurses to be a higher type woman of superior education, and the necessity for her not to simply care for the sick but also to teach the laws of cleanliness.[39]

A lively discussion immediately followed the papers on district nursing and was reconvened again later that week at the invitation of the president of the VNA of Chicago, Mrs. E. C. Dudley. Thus for the first time—and, for many, presumably the last time—American district nurses and their supporters had the opportunity to discuss at length with the English founders of the field the pressing issues faced by all.[40]

One can reasonably assume that the papers and subsequent discussions strongly influenced the development of district nursing in this country. Probably one of those most affected by these proceedings was Lillian Wald, who would prove to be the creative shaper of the field. Wald attended the congress having already decided to abandon her studies at the Women's Medical College of the New York Infirmary for what she considered the more worthwhile work of tending the nursing needs of the sick poor. With the help of her friend and fellow nurse Mary Brewster, she planned to move to the Lower East Side of New York the next month, determined to put into practice the Nightingale and Craven conception of nursing she had studied during her training at the New

York Hospital. The Henry Street Nurses' Settlement was the immediate consequence, but Wald's influence would go far beyond nursing.[41]

The following June, Hampton married physician Hunter Robb and moved
with him to Cleveland. There she remained active in local nursing affairs, serving on the executive committee of the Cleveland VNA from its founding in
1901 until her accidental death in 1910.[42] By the time of Hampton's death,
the Cleveland association had already become one of the more important and
influential organizations in the field.[43] Dock left Baltimore in the summer of
1893 to take over the Illinois Training School in Chicago and then, after a short
vacation at home, joined Wald at Henry Street in 1896.[44] Here, according to one
biographer, "her benign socialist tendencies were absorbed in practical philanthropy." But even after the departures of Dock and Hampton, district nursing
remained highly esteemed at Hopkins. Early graduates of Hopkins became the
leading visiting nurses in this country: Anne Stevens, Ada Carr, Ellen La Motte,
Mary Lent, Elizabeth Fox, Alta Dines, Florence Patterson, Yssabella Waters,
and Katharine Olmstead.[45]

Hampton was followed as superintendent at Hopkins by her new assistant and Hopkins graduate Adelaide Nutting. Like her predecessor, Nutting had
always been interested in visiting nurse work. Later, when Nutting left Baltimore to direct the institutional administration and nursing education program
at Teachers College, Columbia University, she was able to further develop what
would prove a lifelong association with both Dock and Wald. Their shared
interests in finding the means to prepare graduate nurses for the demands of
visiting nursing would shape many developments within the field.[46]

IV

While off to a laudable start, visiting nursing remained a rather small enterprise
at the time of the World's Fair, conducted in a total of thirty-five associations by
no more than sixty-five nurses. But this would not long remain the case, for the
visiting nurse had been introduced during a time of social, medical, and demographic transformation that would greatly enhance the demand for her services.
As a result, VNAs, charity organizations, parish churches, hospitals, and even
industries all began hiring trained nurses to meet their special needs. With this
work being taken up by such a diverse array of organizations, the somewhat
restrictive designation "district nurse" began to be replaced by the more generic
title, "visiting nurse."[47]

Usually, after only a brief interval of tension, the dispensary and private
physicians who cared for the sick poor in their homes came to appreciate the
contribution these nurses had to make. They soon demonstrated their ability

to relieve these physicians of a great deal of responsibility for the regular care of indigent patients. Their aptitude for bringing order and cleanliness, albeit often temporary, to the homes of the sick poor seemed to assure a more favorable outcome and made the task of giving care more pleasant for all involved.[48]

Another factor contributing to the rapid acceptance of the visiting nurse was the rising cost of hospital care and a growing willingness to support any effort that reduced the number of charity patients seeking hospitalization. In their efforts to shed the stigma of their image as a social service for the needy, hospitals valued any program that helped make them appear more attractive. Obviously, one way to relieve hospital burdens—caused by what some contemporary spokesmen asserted was excessive and indiscriminate charity—was to provide the poor with more care in their homes while simultaneously teaching them how to stay healthy.[49]

Thus the visiting nurse, seemingly assured of success, entered the twentieth century with both clear purpose and vision, backed by a strong constituency eager to support what to them appeared an important undertaking from any point of view. Since the work would clearly continue to grow, a major concern for those already in the field was finding an adequate supply of the right kind of nurse.

Because the visiting nurse often found herself working alone, the most basic requirement was for her to have trained in a large general hospital that provided a wide range of clinical experiences. But while almost any woman could learn the necessary "theories, systems and methods," few possessed the other essential qualifications required for this type of work. In district nursing, claimed one authority on the subject, "more than in any other branch of the profession, a nurse 'should be born, not made.'" The essential characteristic that no amount of hospital work could cultivate was, of course, the natural gift of personality. Personality in the case of the visiting nurse meant tact, gentleness, sympathy, ingenuity, resourcefulness, and firmness.[50]

More was required because visiting nursing was never simply good bedside nursing. No longer was the nurse's sole concern a patient in a clean bed in a nice clean ward. Suddenly, explained one nurse, she would enter the patient's home and discover that the home and family life of her patient were as important as his diet or treatment. While the doctor diagnosed a disease, she came to understand that she must diagnose the whole situation. Used to taking orders, she must learn to convince others over whom she had no authority to follow her directions. It was at this point that "personality" would presumably make all the difference in outcome. If successful, the good visiting nurse would be capable of making do with the meager resources found in the home, creating an environment conducive to the patient's recovery while simultaneously coaxing or reasoning the family into its maintenance in her absence.

But gaining the friendship and confidence of families in her care was only the beginning of the visiting nurse's job. She was also expected to be able to go out into the community and make herself known to other families, to find patients and not simply to wait for patients to find her. Finally, she needed "personality" because meeting her patients' complex medical and social needs meant being able to work in harmony with other charitable organizations as well as with the doctors in her district.[51] As one nurse suggested, the ideal visiting nurse was a faultless creature "possessing all the virtues, combining the experience of age with the enthusiasm of youth and also having a sense of humor, which is perhaps the only thing which will make the years" of this kind of work possible.[52]

Many nurses, while attracted to visiting work, found it too mentally and physically exhausting to pursue. Walking long distances in all kinds of weather, climbing endless flights of stairs, cleaning and disinfecting patients' rooms, changing beds, and constant exposure to disease were all part of the visiting nurses' daily routine. While the "delicate" nurse found this an impossible undertaking, even the strongest found themselves exhausted at the end of such a day. Some were simply too revolted by the filth, vermin, and dirt typical of overcrowded tenements. Exhausted, discouraged, and not infrequently sick, many nurses left for more lucrative or easier work, while others left to marry or were called home because of death or illness in the family. As a result, the turnover on many staffs was high, while replacements were often difficult to find.[53]

While not all nurses were fit for visiting nursing, not all homebound, indigent patients required these services. Such an undertaking was not only impossible; it was also unnecessary.[54] To survive, suggested one nurse, you must conserve your own "force and not recklessly scatter [your] time, strength, and service." The wise nurse, she concluded, followed the dictum "a few patients well treated [was] more satisfactory than many just cursorily looked after."[55] Thus underlying her work must be "a stratum of strong good sense" that enabled the nurse to accurately determine which cases to follow and which to avoid. Climbing five flights of stairs with a full day of serious cases awaiting her only to find the patient away or "incorrigible" was usually the only lesson required to teach most nurses which patients to bequeath to the sole care of the doctor.[56]

It was also the nurse's responsibility to identify those patients that "properly" belonged in the hospital rather than at home—and on her caseload. According to Wald, the patient's condition, duration of illness, financial situation, and home environment were the criteria used by doctors and nurses in the "shifting process." Examples of cases better cared for in the hospital were "brain troubles" where quiet surroundings were demanded, contagious diseases that would endanger the family and tenement because isolation too often proved impossible, operations requiring aseptic conditions, and fractures and injuries requiring apparatus not available at home. On average, only about 10 percent of visiting nurses' cases seemed to end up in the hospital.[57]

Having carefully avoided the "comparatively worthless cases" and those better cared for in the hospital, what remained was, as one VNA suggested, "our legitimate work."[58] While Wald claimed that any patient in bed needed a visiting nurse, other interpretations were a bit more cautious.[59] The Philadelphia Visiting Nurse Society (VNS), for example, saw chronic complaints, such as cancer and rheumatism; sudden acute illness; slight accidents; "diseases of dirt," such as bedsores; and maternity cases as within their appropriate realm.[60] During seasons of "comparative neighborhood healthfulness," the nurse's domain was often extended to include the follow-up of minor illness among children, the teaching of family hygiene and simple nutritious cookery, and showing mothers how to keep their children clean and free from vermin.[61] But even within these seemingly compatible visions, few could agree on the relative value of actual nursing care as opposed to education of the patients' families. By 1904, the proper balance of these two activities had already become and would remain for years an unresolvable issue.[62]

Statistics presented in many annual reports suggest in more detail who the nurses' patients were and the problems they treated. Boston's IDNA kept some of the best data during this early period, and their experience appears typical of those encountered by most larger VNAs. In Boston, prior to 1910, the vast majority of the visiting nurses' patients were women (40 percent) and children (43 percent). While most (70 percent) patients were treated for acute medical problems, 14 percent had chronic problems, 11 percent were surgical patients, and only 2 percent were obstetrical cases. Most patients were discharged as "well" or "improved," while only a small percentage (5 percent) continued to need care. Finally, less than 5 percent were "discharged by death."[63]

A host of these patients were immigrants—mainly Irish, Italian, and Russian—whose language the nurses did not understand and whose customs were familiar only, as one nurse suggested, when daily encounters made them unavoidable. Their "national ideas," those handed down from "grandmother to mother to child," made the nurse's work inordinately complex. More comfortable relying on "superstitious observation and charms," the patients often reacted to the nurse as a "most cruel and unfeeling monster" and to her hygienic message with hostility.[64]

The nurses' perceptions of their patients were often conveyed in a "nurse's story," which formed an essential part of most annual reports. Used, no doubt, as propaganda to ensure financial support for the agency, they conveyed a consistent image. In these stories, nurses described their patients as more or less dependent, ignorant, improperly nourished, and on occasion, shiftless and intemperate. Their homes were portrayed as small, overcrowded, poorly ventilated rooms where—according to one typical annual report—"the dirt of many years has accumulated and where the absence of cleanliness, while deplored, finds some excuse for its non-existence." Disregarding the most ordinary rules of hygiene, even during illness, they were seen as living in "such unwholesome circumstances" that when "stricken" by disease, their recovery was "either not to be hoped for, or at best very slow and unsatisfactory."[65] Not surprisingly, many "nurse stories" stressed the danger created for the rest of the population by these patients. For example, one story described a woman who worked in a candy store and was found by the nurse to have tuberculosis. The need for the visiting nurse was, of course, dramatized by the accompanying warning: "Think of all the tuberculosis bacilli presented with each package of candy."[66]

No matter what their overall perception of their patients, visiting nurses found many of their habits peculiar. Feeding dill pickles or pork chops to infants was seen as shocking, while practices such as wrapping infants in long bands "to keep them straight" or fears of opening windows at night were seen as simply "ignorant." In some instances, they described their patients' behavior as not only incomprehensible but life-threatening as well. One story published in the *Visiting Nurse Quarterly* (*VNQ*), for example, told of parents who, having taken their sick baby to the doctor, failed to give either treatment or medicine because the baby was "too much sick." Leaving the infant "untouched, uncared for, in a very dirty cradle," to the dismay of the nurse, they had instead covered the baby with the warm blood of a chicken and then tied the bird's legs to a chair. This superstitious act was reported, it was claimed, to demonstrate the immigrants' "great need of education"—that is, the visiting nurse.[67]

Whatever she actually encountered in the homes of her patients, the nurse rarely found herself alone, for neighbors were always an integral part of any visit. It was inevitable, explained Wald, that "the flock of neighbors" would appear drawn by "curiosity, idleness, interest or sympathy." "Firmly dismissing the curious and idle," the nurse often found it helpful to accept the help of "any intelligent person" who might appear. Often forced to rely on a neighborly interpreter, many nurses felt that much of the "enthusiasm, force and personality" of their message was often lost in the process. This was particularly true, claimed one nurse, "if the interpreter happens to be a neighbor who has had eleven children of her own," even if they all had died.[68]

On the surface, tenement slums and immigrants appeared to create an unstable and uncontrollable situation, but to the competent visiting nurse, this was simply a "large outdoor hospital." The nurse's district was, she claimed, her ward where she directed and supervised patient care. Like the hospital, each district had its system of bedside notes, case records, and established etiquette among physician, nurse, and patient. Of course, unlike the hospital, the nurse more often found herself in charge.[69]

Most visiting nurses worked six days a week, making only emergency visits on Sunday. They made between eight and twelve visits on a normal day and stayed in each home for one-half to two hours depending on the severity of the problem. Most patients received an average of eight to ten visits before they were discharged.[70] A typical day would begin at 8:00 a.m. with visits to the patients considered "dangerously ill." Similarly, the day would conclude eight to ten hours later with a return visit to these same patients. The rest of the day was devoted to the care of patients with such problems as varicose ulcers, bronchitis, fevers of various origins, abscesses, a few "chronics," and an assortment of infectious diseases. Good nursing care was thought to include keeping the air in the room fresh and wholesome and the patient, patient's bed, and sick room clean and quiet; establishing regularity in the giving of nourishment and medicines, skillfully observing the patient's condition, carefully recorded or communicated to the doctor; and taking appropriate measures to prevent the spread of contagious diseases.[71]

Much of the nurses' efforts focused on what was described as alleviating patients' distressing symptoms through the use of an armamentarium that included glycerin for parched lips, cold compresses or ice bags for headache, and weak mustard plaster or a little bruised mint wilted in brandy over the stomach for vomiting. Fever patients were treated with a "temperature bath" and a cool atmosphere created by pouring cold water on the floor or by hanging sheets rung out in ice water around the room. Patients with bronchitis or pneumonia received similar care but additionally had their chests rubbed with camphorated oil and were then placed in a cotton jacket or had their chests covered with hot flannel. Rheumatic joints were bandaged and children with measles bathed in saleratus water, while the danger of contagious disease was abated by the hanging of sheets dipped in a carbolic solution.[72]

All this, plus certain basic emergency interventions, was taught to either the family or a neighbor to be carried out in the nurse's absence. Finally, visiting nurses were not infrequently called upon to treat their patients' family pets.

One canary with asthma was cured by a change in climate (removal from a smoky kitchen), while in another instance, the nurse claimed to have successfully treated a monkey with measles. For the visiting nurse, healing the sick and spreading the gospel of cleanliness could not be narrowly confined.[73]

By the end of the century, what had begun twenty years before as a self-conscious copy of English models was evolving into something rather different. While the English had established a well-standardized national system of district nursing, Americans were more inclined to have their visiting nurses carry on this work in a variety of ways. Although support developed slowly at first, the nurses and their lady sponsors were confident that they had found the best means "at the smallest cost" for helping the "conditions of the poor, sick or well." With a growing number of immigrants, the ever-present danger of contagious diseases, and changes in the functions of the hospital, others began to share their views. Quickly, the image of the visiting nurse "dispelling and purifying . . . the darkness, disease, and foul air of the tenements" took on both symbolic and practical appeal. Eventually, the growing popularity of the visiting nurse would mean more services, therapeutic and preventive, for the poor. It would also lead to the development of an important new field of employment, one that offered nurses an irresistible combination—economic security and professional independence.[74]

Chapter 2

Creating Their Own Domain

Ladies, Nurses, and the Sick Poor

On a cold winter morning in 1902, Mrs. Isabel Lowman, the wife of a prominent physician and a member of the Board of Trustees of the Visiting Nurse
Association (VNA) of Cleveland, agreed to accompany one of the association's
nurses on her rounds: "I shall always remember my surprise . . . ," she recalled
ten years later, "at the situation we encountered in the first home. . . . I sat in a
rocking chair, feeling very low in spirit and quite benumbed by astonishment
and a kind of terror."[1]

In contrast, the nurse, who was young, attractive, neat, and dainty in
appearance, seemed to Mrs. Lowman quite at home. While Mrs. Lowman sat,
presumably trying to overcome her shock, the nurse "attacked the situation
with cheerfulness and decision," rapidly setting the sick room and sick patient
in order, washing the patient, changing the bed, combing her hair, and reordering the room for proper ventilation and light. She determined the patient's condition and left notes for the physician when he returned. Finally, the "gossipy
old woman" neighbor was replaced by a "sensible looking" one who promised
to carry out the nurse's instructions.[2]

They made two more visits together before Mrs. Lowman reached the end of
her endurance. Finding herself "tired, cold, and a little frightened" at the scenes
into which her "young guide" had led her, she returned home. The nurse, who
in contrast to Mrs. Lowman seemed entirely competent to handle these "terrible
situations," proceeded her way to visit the six or seven patients remaining on
her list.[3]

Mrs. Lowman's recounting of her introduction to visiting nursing nicely
illustrates the focus of this chapter: the distinctive yet potentially unstable

nature of the functions of lady managers and nurses prior to World War I. As this apocryphal story suggests, differences between these two groups were not confined simply to areas of professional competence but reflected social class as well. Since nurses were not ladies and ladies were not nurses, their mutual dependence seemed obvious. Because of their unique training, visiting nurses were a most practical means of caring for the sick poor at home. The lady managers, on the other hand, were uniquely qualified to find and manage the money needed to pay the nurses.

This symbiotic relationship remained stable enough until 1909 or 1910 when, according to Mary Gardner (a prominent visiting nurse), "popularity struck." With it came a growing demand for visiting nurses not only to care for the sick but to do preventive work with babies, mothers, schoolchildren, and patients with tuberculosis.[4] In addition, after 1909, when the Metropolitan Life Insurance Company (MLI) began paying for nursing visits to its sick policy-holders, VNAs also provided more services to the working class.

The lady managers, eager to help launch these new fields, found that their enthusiasm exceeded their ability to finance and manage agency growth. Not surprisingly, with expansion came chaos for many agencies: the result of large staffs of thirty to forty nurses, four or five divergent new programs, a mélange of agreements with other voluntary agencies, and recurring budget deficits. But what seemed chaotic to managers appeared to be an exciting new future to nurses. This rapid growth meant more services to the poor immediately and might lead ultimately to the development of important new fields of employment. Eventually, both lady managers and nurses would be forced to realize the inevitability of radical organization of visiting nursing.[5]

I

In 1900, there were only 115 organizations, employing a total of 130 visiting nurses.[6] All the associations were small; many had no headquarters at all, while others used a backroom or possibly a spare corner in a dispensary. Most were, as one participant later suggested, the "pet charity of a small self-limited group of lady bountifuls."[7] In these associations, the lady managers dominated all matters from general policy and fundraising to the most petty decisions.

Women were sought as members of the board of managers for a variety of reasons, and not all were expected to be active on a regular basis.[8] All boards required some wealthy members who could be counted on to support the organization and some members with social connections who would help with fundraising. Male board membership was usually limited to the financial or advisory committees, whose functions were to ensure a positive relationship with the community's business, medical, and philanthropic interests. Men were expected to provide money, prestige, and advice, not time. As Annie Brainard, member of the Cleveland board put it, members of this type were figureheads for the association, "representing the highest thought and spirit of the community."[9]

The real work was done by a small group of women, those with sufficient leisure time and interest to keep the association alive. These women were members of the executive committee and the lady managers responsible for the supervision of the nurses. Most VNAs had an executive committee of four or five women who worked regularly and were given the authority to decide any question arising between monthly board meetings. The ladies responsible for supervising the nurses frequently modeled their work after the English system by dividing the city into districts with a nurse and two managers assigned to each district. The nurse and her lady managers would meet weekly to review the nurse's work.[10]

By all accounts the relationship between the nurses and managers was intensely personal, the result, no doubt, of their weekly meetings. Here the nurse would serve as an ambassador, as Mary Beard (a visiting nurse) put it, between "one group in society to another group very removed from it."[11] This process was said to have a "corrective influence," helping the heretofore sheltered ladies develop true wisdom and a sympathetic relationship with those whose lives were perplexed by ignorance, poverty, and disease.[12] In exchange, the nurse was given an opportunity to review her cases with women who had seen a very different side of life—whose cleanliness, morality, and good housekeeping were exemplary. Through their "personal oversight," the ladies provided an uplifting effect on the nurse's practice by helping her pay painstaking attention to every detail.[13]

Despite such assumptions of mutual dependence, there was little social or professional equality between the nurses and the managers. As Katharine Tucker observed, "Most often their relationship followed the English distinction between the leisure class and working class. The workers were regarded somewhat as clerks or office boys to do the bidding of the board."[14] Not only did the ladies see themselves as socially superior to the nurses; they also expected the nurses to defer to their judgment in professional nursing matters.[15]

Even in agencies large enough to require a head nurse, the managers were still clearly in charge. For example, in 1887, Philadelphia hired a head nurse, Miss Haydock, to "be in charge of all those employed by the society."[16] The next year, she was given a larger salary because of her growing responsibilities, which now included supervising the nurses, "the helpers," the work, and the office business and teaching the students.[17] But these broad responsibilities were destined to be rapidly eroded. By May 1888, several ladies had been appointed to the nurses' committee to "superintend the nurses directly, to pay them monthly, and as far as possible to ration their work."[18] Within a month, the committee, which did not include Haydock, had created a set of rules for the nurses, which dealt with personal cleanliness and behavior, hours of work, records, duties of the head nurse, and the monthly meetings between nurses and managers.[19] The rules were presented to the nurses without objection. At the same meeting, the managers made clear their intention of increasing their control and moved to reduce that of the head nurse by announcing that Haydock should decide only unimportant cases and leave "the disposition of more doubtful ones to the committee on nurses."[20]

Still not completely satisfied that they were maintaining adequate control over the staff, the board decided it would be best to have the nurses live in the house, the administrative center of the society, "under the charge of an experienced matron and under the constant supervision of the managers."[21] The board announced their decision to the nurses realizing that some would not accept the proposal and would have to be replaced. As anticipated, "the result was much distress and confusion in the staff and much turnover."[22] Although Haydock was asked to stay on under the "new regulations" in any position she wanted, she declined the offer, thus terminating the first experiment with a head nurse for the Philadelphia Visiting Nurse Society (VNS).[23]

A year later, Philadelphia was still without "an efficient head nurse." The ladies were clearly in charge.[24] By July 1890, they had created an even more restrictive set of rules for the nurses. It is not clear whether the new rules were developed in response to some specific incident involving the staff or simply reflected the ladies' fears of how the nurses might behave. The new rules required the nurses to treat patients with utmost gentleness, to work when on duty, to accept no liquor from patients, and to be neat. In addition, a set of house rules was provided, specifying everything from hours for meals and visitors to when to turn out the lights.[25]

For those nurses who failed to comply with the rules or who, in the judgment of the managers, failed to provide appropriate care, the most common recourse was dismissal. Nurses were asked to resign for a variety of reasons ranging from an unpleasant personality to unsatisfactory performance.[26] On one occasion, a nurse complained about the Philadelphia board's decision to let her go, claiming her dismissal had been on personal grounds. The board investigated her charges and concluded that, just as she had claimed, she had not neglected her patient but dismissed her instead for "incompetence."

Displeased by the whole affair, it took steps to prevent its recurrence by ruling "that the form of dismissal of every nurse be dictated by the board and that each nurse be engaged with the understanding that if she is dismissed as not being suited to the work, no further reason shall be asked."[27] The board had learned its lesson and would not be distracted by attacks on its authority.

Dismissal was apparently not an uncommon form of education for young visiting nurses. Gardner—a member of a prominent Providence, Rhode Island, family, the first head nurse of that city's visiting nurse society, and a prolific writer of both fiction and nonfiction—frequently chose the precarious relationship between nurses and their board as a theme in her writings.[28] In *Katharine Kent*, her first novel, she described a young nurse much as she later described herself, as lacking knowledge and experience but "eager to blaze a trail."[29] In the novel, Katharine's enthusiasm hampered her success in her first job because, failing to recognize the value and knowledge of the board members, she acted without regard for their opinions. This wisdom was acquired only through much self-searching and after the board decided to replace her with an older nurse. A family friend later comforted Katharine: "There is nothing in your story that spells permanent disaster but there is a good deal that must be changed before you can hope to achieve success or carry your work into a better future."[30]

Miss A. E. Beer, the first superintendent hired by the Instructive District Nursing Association (IDNA) of Boston would probably have told a similar story. She was hired in May 1900 by the board to "see that the best work was done and to understand the relative working condition of each district."[31] Beer approached her assignment with enthusiasm and by November had visited each nurse, reviewed their record books, and listened to their oral reports. Her summary to the board made all too clear numerous problems. She did not approve of the nurses' cotton bags, which she felt were unsuitable for district work; she found the office closets were dusty and not systematic; and she thought record books were not neatly kept and the aprons were dirty. Nor was she very impressed with the staff, especially their lack of attention "to the details of district nursing and in some cases their personal appearance." Some were careless about disinfecting their hands, and some were "Sallies too old to do justice to the work." She even suggested that the society's agreement to send nurses to accompany the dispensary doctors on their morning rounds was a waste of time.[32] Beer's impressions and recommendations were ignored by the board, and she resigned to get married the next year. She was replaced by Martha Stark. Stark, already a member of the staff, apparently had the ability to supervise the staff and the wisdom to avoid criticizing long-standing traditions. In contrast to Beer, her stay with the association lasted eleven years.[33]

Apparently, a staff of twelve nurses, a business office, and often a nurse's home required more managing than most lady managers were willing or able to sustain. The most frequent solution was to hire someone, either a head nurse or matron, to supervise the staff daily. But the ladies quickly found they had difficulty relinquishing control of any aspect of the work and frequently became overbearing in their struggles to find an appropriate balance of managerial control. On the other hand, inexperienced head nurses, through their excessive enthusiasm and criticism, often gave the appearance of disregard for past work and frequently antagonized the board. Compromise was uncommon; either the head nurse conformed to the will of the board or left to be replaced by someone more cooperative.

II

But the problems of most VNAs would not remain the sole domain of the lady managers for much longer. As the staff grew and new programs were initiated, both internal and external relationships began to go awry. Record systems seemed inadequate, supervision superficial, and programs overspecialized; no matter how reluctantly, the lady managers were forced to recognize that their creations had become so inefficient as to require radical reorganization.[34]

Most boards, realizing it was no longer plausible or possible to attempt to oversee the initiation of this new order, sought professional help. Management of their organization would become the responsibility of a new kind of superintendent, women "of unusual training, splendid endorsement, and courage."[35] In fact, these new superintendents did differ significantly from their predecessors. Well-educated, often college graduates, they came from good families and could be trusted by the ladies, as one Boston manager suggested, to take "hold of their problems . . . with a sympathetic understanding of the past and a clear vision of the possibilities for the future."[36]

Despite the perceived necessity for these changes, some feared the lady managers' lack of daily involvement would produce a growing sense of estrangement on the part of the nurses. Might the staff, queried an older Cleveland manager, come to see them as those "well-fed, well-housed, and well-warmed" managers who "hold the pursestrings and count out the dole?"[37] Just as surely, she believed the lady managers were doomed to experience a kind of spiritual anemia, as well as indignation, at being "relegated to a role where one's money is thought more useful and desirable than oneself."[38]

But city by city, a pattern of reorganization and redefinition of authority was repeated. In Boston, it was accomplished by Beard; in Providence, by Gardner; in Chicago, by Edna Foley; first in Dayton and later in Washington, DC, by Elizabeth Fox;[39] in Baltimore and Los Angeles, by Mary Lent; and in Philadelphia, by Tucker.[40] That the outcomes were fairly consistent is not surprising, since this "ring of women," as Gardner called them, regularly exchanged ideas and experiences.[41] This same network of nurses would, in 1912, form the National Organization for Public Health Nursing (NOPHN) to promote similar developments nationwide.[42]

Not surprisingly, the issues addressed and the solutions eventually sought by these nursing associations were similar to those confronted by the voluntary hospital. Charles Rosenberg, Morris Vogel, and David Rosner have all discussed this period of transformation, which they suggest was initiated prior to the turn of the century.[43] In contrast, probably because they were smaller and therefore less complex in both an administrative and a financial sense, VNAs did not initiate this process until after 1910.[44] The IDNA of Boston was one of the first to reorganize and will be considered in detail because it typifies the changes that occurred in many VNAs immediately prior to the First World War.

The first inkling that the lady managers of the Boston association shared any concern about their methods occurred in February 1908 when Elizabeth Cordner, a member of the board, requested Boston physician Dr. Hugh Cabot's suggestions about their nursing associations. Cabot began his five-page response by reminding the ladies that any association dependent upon private contributions must be in the position to ensure that no one could question that the work was of the highest attainable standard. This, he believed, was achieved through careful, constant supervision. Unfortunately, he concluded that it seemed "in some respects the supervision of the nurses of your Association was ineffective." He failed to see how ladies meeting with the nurses to discuss cases known only by name constituted the searching inquiry of a semi-medical character essential to good work. Although he realized the association had a superintendent, Stark, who was in charge of the nurses, he could not find any evidence that any kind of strict supervision had been done over the past few years. As for Stark, he concluded, "I should not expect her to do such work as well as other parts of the work which she finds more congenial."[45] But it should be remembered that it was for this purpose precisely that the ladies hired Stark in the first place.

Cabot suggested that the most efficient supervision would be obtained if the ladies hired a superintendent of considerable experience and ability in the field, who would give her whole time to overseeing the nurses' work. Since this would involve an expenditure of money, which the board might hesitate to make, he suggested alternatively obtaining the services of several young medical men "whose business it would be to make rounds with the nurses at frequent, though unknown, intervals and report directly to the Board of Managers." Since these gentlemen would undoubtedly have weight with the community, Cabot felt they would make the work of raising funds easier, granting they found that the work was being done with the greatest possible efficiency.[46]

Not sharing Cabot's assessment of their methods, the ladies found other matters more important. During the next three years, they were preoccupied as their staff grew from fifteen to forty-three people and with the corresponding increase in their budget, from $27,000 to $49,000. New business arrangements were negotiated with the MLI; the maternity program was expanded to include prenatal care; programs in contagion, day nurseries, and industrial nursing were initiated; and finally, their new training school for district nurses was expanding.[47]

But by 1911, the ladies were forced to examine the outcome of these new programs. Visiting nursing was no longer confined to the seven specialized programs of the IDNA; both the Baby Hygiene Association and the city had their own staff of nurses. In fact, among these three groups, families were potentially liable to visits from up to ten different visiting nurses. The managers were forced to conclude that "there are today too many unrelated groups of nurses in Boston. Among them there is much duplication, waste of time and money, and the public, which we are trying to help, is in reality the sufferer."[48]

Michael Davis, director of the Boston Dispensary, shared the managers' concerns that the nurses' work had become too specialized. He believed specialization produced the highest efficiency only when workers "are under a strong, broad and intelligent supervision and when the specialists have a good background of training behind their particular skill."[49] He reminded the ladies that otherwise the result was a number of specialists working more or less independently without the proper correlation. Not only was this a waste of time; it would also fail to affect the desired results. According to Davis, what was needed first was a more authoritative, centralized organization and, at least for a time, less specialization. Eventually, he thought, the managers should hire "a higher type personality or at least provide more training of the rank and file worker."[50]

At last, the lady managers agreed with their critics and were ready to reorganize.[51] In February 1911, they began a search for the right nurse to implement their plan, which eventually incorporated Cabot's and Davis's ideas of professional supervision, centralization, and training. The lady managers felt that their plan was more than the solution to a simple local problem; they were convinced it would serve as a national example.[52] But their search for a new superintendent immediately encountered difficulty, and before it was over a year later, the Boston managers had been turned down by some of the most innovative leaders in the field: Ida Cannon, Foley, Ella Crandall, and Ellen LaMotte.[53]

That the board would choose to vigorously pursue someone like LaMotte suggests either a desire to create a totally new order or, perhaps, their desperation. In either case, their persistence seems surprising. At the time, LaMotte was the only woman department head at the Baltimore Health Department. Although letters of reference consistently praised her unsurpassed ability to handle difficult situations, her quickness of mind, her power of literally expression, and her original ideas, they all ended on a cautionary note, suggesting, in essence, that the same qualities that made LaMotte one of the ablest women in the nursing profession might not be totally acceptable to the Boston board. Their concern included her very pronounced character and strong opinions, her tendency to become bored, careless, and indifferent if the work became routine, and the possibility that she might want to do everything the Hopkins way. Finally, she was known to be "a rabid suffragist."[54] The board, apparently willing to take their chances, offered LaMotte the job. But she was unwilling to leave her Baltimore position, feeling it was still in too unsettled a state. The board, unconvinced, tried again, but she again declined their offer.

Finally, in November of 1919, Crandall recommended Beard for the job, but the managers hesitated, apparently sharing Beard's concern about her "unpreparedness" for undertaking such "a big social and nursing cause."[55] Since no one "better fitted" was at hand, however, both were forced to give the matter further consideration. Crandall assured the board that Beard was the right person for Boston, but then again, Crandall was eager to see the position filled and thus save herself any "repeated solicitations" from the managers.[56] No matter what her motivations were, Crandall did claim to be very impressed with Beard, "her appearance, voice, manner, mental attitude, and mental grasp" and especially the fact that she was a "New England lady born and bred."[57]

In actuality, Beard did have several years of experience as a head nurse with the Waterbury, Connecticut, VNA. Rev. John Lewis, president of that association, felt that on the whole, Beard would be well-suited for the Boston position because of her real ability, self-confidence, and personal charm. He noted that she did much better when in command than as a subordinate, that she managed other people's work better than her own, and that she was not a good financier or good at keeping accounts. Finally, he assured the board that if she had a secretary, she would do admirably, adding equivocally that "she needs one."[58]

When Beard began her new position in February 1912, she was confronted with twenty-five years of tradition, twenty-seven lady managers whose expectations included the elevation of their association to "its proper place in the community and the country," and forty-nine nurses caught in the middle.[59] By April, she had initiated a plan of reorganization, which resulted in so complete a change as to produce an institutional revolution. Although most of the nurses remained on the staff, some found it difficult, as Beard put it, to "fall in loyally with the changes."[60]

Beard's plan called for a lumping together of the work being done by the various nurses so that each would no longer specialize in one type of problem but would become a general practitioner—what she called a "neighborhood" or "community" nurse. Consistent with this neighborhood plan, seven branch stations were created, each with a supervisor to do the "executive work," advising, and supervision and a staff of nurses to meet any health need that might arise in the neighborhood.[61]

Beard envisioned the nurse as a community consultant for families, "where illness has produced poor living conditions or those in which poor living conditions have produced illness."[62] Eventually, she predicted, "all the people of a neighborhood, regardless of income, would employ our nurses, and each patient so cared for will feel a personal responsibility to raise the money necessary . . . in order to supply all the nursing the community requires."[63] If successful, this plan would shift the focus of visiting nursing from the sick poor to the whole community. Thus at last free of the stigma of charity, the visiting nurse would become not only the neighborhood's nurse but the only nurse in the neighborhood.[64]

Recognizing that much "educational work" was required before the association could get away from the "old charity idea," Beard decided to use a strategy certain to attract attention. She changed the nurses' uniforms, believing that in areas where the staff were familiar figures, this would advertise the fact that the association was now doing neighborhood nursing. The principle of collecting a fee, however small, was emphasized, and the association's "scale of prices," ranging from nothing to fifty cents a visit, was conscientiously advertised. Finally, a more "scientific" and accurate method of keeping records was established, making it possible to better document the good work being done as well as the relationship of their work to the national public health problems.[65]

During her second year with the association, Beard's major concern was the upgrading of the staff by replacing all the temporary nurses with twenty-two new nurses who had completed a postgraduate course in public health nursing. The replacements, she assured the board, "want to do this sort of nursing more than any other work, are full of enthusiasm and have made sacrifices to obtain a special education for it."[66] Despite these rather dramatic alterations in the staff, Beard was pleased with the outcome. By 1915, she reported that the nurses had become responsible, independent authorities and the amount of work done had increased.[67]

All that remained was the updating of the "Rules for the Nurses" and the creation of written standards describing the proper techniques for each type of nursing care. These standards would be used to grade the nurses, thus assuring the elimination of waste and the most efficient fulfillment of the association's ends.[68]

At last the plan was completed, and naturally, it too would be graded. It was important, according to Beard, to be willing to test one's efforts and results with courage and a sincere desire to learn the truth, either positive or negative. Such a test should first make comparisons, second determine if any historic developments had been achieved, and finally, analyze and study the work in relation to past achievements and future needs.[69]

The formation of the NOPHN made the "test by comparison," as Beard put it, "both delightful and easy," for at the annual meetings they could talk with representatives from VNAs from across the country and Canada. Beard, Mrs. Codman (a board member), and four staff nurses attended the first meeting, which was held in Atlantic City in June 1913. Not surprisingly, they found that many shared their concerns about standards, records, statistics, and the need to extend their work to "all people."[70]

Although Beard suggested in the *Annual Report* for 1913 that, as she remembered it, the central idea expressed at these meetings was that of neighborhood nursing, few other reports of the convention shared her recollections.[71] In fact, Boston's official decision to abandon specialization in favor of a generalized service placed them at the forefront of a debate that continued unresolved for years.[72] But on the whole, the comparison proved favorable. The Boston association had clearly attained a position of prominence.

Beard ranked neighborhood nursing as an important contribution to public health nursing and chose to interpret the fees collected as an appropriate index of success. Consistent with this criterion, she included a "fee study" in her annual reports but left it to the reader to determine if these results indicated success or failure.[73] Based on Beard's data and criteria, most readers would probably have concluded that neighborhood nursing had not been a great success—since the percent of patients paying fees had remained stable at roughly 24 percent.[74] Data available in the treasurer's reports suggest that a somewhat more positive picture was achieved, as the percent of total budget received from fees increased from 3 percent ($1,521) the year prior to reorganization to 9 percent ($6,333) by 1915.[75]

In terms of productivity, on the other hand, neighborhood nursing was clearly a success. Between 1911 and 1915, the number of visits made during a year increased by 15 percent (16,922), and the number of patients receiving care increased by 41 percent (4,100), while only three nurses were added to the staff.[76] For each nurse, this increase meant caring for ninety-eight more patients a year. In a financial sense, the outcome was not entirely positive because the nurses, who were better educated and working harder, were also better paid. But this additional $17,000 in wages seemed to cause the managers little distress.[77] In fact, the board consistently encouraged Beard's plans for expansion, reassuring her from the onset that they planned to "think in terms of work rather than money."[78] Although they assured her the money would be there to do the work, they incurred, and eventually covered, a deficit of about $3,000 each year.[79]

Thus at the end of four years, Beard, with the support of the board, had created a profoundly different organization. Changed was their approach to financial support, from total dependence on donations toward the patient as a source of income. Gone were the lady managers' naive business practices, replaced by the more professional approach of nurses committed to eliminating waste, maintaining reliable records, and consistently producing the highest quality of nursing care. But most dramatic was the altered relationship between managers and nurses. For as the nurses came to dominate, the managers retired into the background to such an extent that the supervisors began to complain that they no longer knew even the names of the managers.[80] Boston was only the first of many such transformations.

III

Even prior to this period of rapid expansion, the financial status of most VNAs was never very secure, and deficits of a few thousand dollars regularly recurred.[81] But a little overspending was of much less concern to lady managers than a large balance in the treasury. Underspending was for them "a confession of failure in as much as it represents just that much more work undone."[82] In the same spirit, annual budgets were based on community demand for nursing service and financed through donations, subscriptions, revenues from dinners or tag days, endowments, and to a lesser extent, payment from patients. When the managers inevitably found themselves in what Gardner called the "rather embarrassing position of a man who had suddenly set up a large establishment without any particular increase in income," they fortunately could go to their friends who would rally to their support.[83]

This technique ran few risks for agencies with small budgets, but by 1912, many of the larger VNAs had annual budgets of over $50,000.[84] At this level of spending, it became increasingly difficult for the ladies to raise sufficient funds and "appalling deficits" became more common.[85] Not surprisingly, some managers described themselves as having "an almost desperate sense of being overwhelmed by the sudden growth and extension of this kind of enterprise which they had helped into being . . . without a correspondingly rapid increase in sources of support."[86]

For many boards of managers, the paying patient increasingly seemed an, as yet, uncultivated means of survival. There were, in fact, according to Gardner, three groups of people to be considered by every VNA.[87] The first class included the aged, chronically ill, widows with children, and others who because of health or other handicaps could never be self-supporting. It was from this group that most of their needy patients came—patients otherwise unable to pay physicians or nursing costs. The second group comprised those with reasonable means, enough to have saved for a rainy day, who could make a small payment for nursing services. Most associations had very early decided to make their services available to this class of "thrifty wage earners" who, they reassured themselves, would not be willing to collect money, "realizing the injustice to the patient of encouraging or allowing him to have for nothing that which he is able or ought to pay." Many agencies found that it was among this class of patients that they obtained their best results.[88] Apparently, patients were not equally eager to avoid being pauperized, since there is mention of having difficulty exacting payments from patients, and in most agencies, very little of the annual budget came from paying patients.[89] The third class of patients included those with incomes placing them well beyond the grasp of poverty but who could not afford a private nurse. This class, as yet virtually unexplored, could certainly benefit from the visits of a nurse during illness and might be expected to pay the full price of a visit.[90]

Actually, after 1909, many VNAs already become the beneficial recipients of substantial financial assistance in their efforts to extend their services to the working class. That was the year that Dr. Lee Frankel founded the welfare division of the MLI to carry on a broad health education program. One of his major concerns was the large amount of illness among policyholders reported by company insurance agents who made regular visits to their homes. It was Wald who suggested to Frankel that this need could be met by sending out visiting nurses.

The mutual advantages were readily apparent. At a cost five cents a policy, the Metropolitan could reduce the number of death benefits it had to pay.

Without additional fundraising, district nursing associations could extend their services to more of the working class. The experiment began in New York, in June of 1909, with the visiting nurses of Henry Street Settlement House and was quickly expanded to include Boston; Baltimore; Washington, DC; Chicago; Cleveland; and St. Louis. By 1911, "Mother Met," as the company was affectionately called, had decided to offer nursing services throughout the entire country. Where possible, it arranged for existing VNAs to provide the care; where that was not possible, it hired its own nurses. Three years after the service was initiated, the Metropolitan was paying for one million nursing visits each year at a cost of roughly $500,000.[91] For many large associations, this arrangement was of substantial financial benefit. For example, the Metropolitan paid for 32 percent of the cases carried by the Philadelphia association in 1911; 33,494 visits made by the Chicago visiting nurses in 1912; and 20 percent of the Providence District Nursing Association's (DNA) budget in 1913.[92]

But the Metropolitan's financial support of visiting nursing was hardly a philanthropic contribution; it was a nosiness investment. Eager to receive the highest possible returns for that investment, they quickly became concerned about many of the VNAs' management practices. Their costs were often too high because the nurses made too few visits each day, the records systems were poor and often inaccurate, and they had not done enough to attract paying patients. The lady managers could hardly disagree, but they found Frankel's solutions less than appealing, since they required drastic alterations in the very nature of their organizations.[93] In his 1913 speech "Visiting Nursing from a Business Organization's Standpoint," he told those attending the first meeting of the NOPHN of his vision of the future. He warned that "if visiting nursing services are to receive the development they should, and are to reach the large mass of the population, less must constantly be laid upon the charitable or philanthropic side." He realized this would be a difficult adjustment, but self-respecting working men and women found any service offered by "the charity nurse" inherently repugnant. Visiting nursing should be conducted as a business proposition and support itself largely from patient payments. These should be made by patients by the visit or annually from employers, fraternal orders, benevolent associations, labor unions, insurance companies, municipalities, or for the poor, by relief agencies.[94]

Visiting nursing could hardly afford to ignore Frankel's opinions, especially when he had privately suggested that his company was considering organizing its own visiting nurse service if the established agencies were not willing to free themselves from this stigma of charity. His ideas were widely discussed, and his speech was even quoted in the annual report of the DNA of

Providence. As Gardner suggested, whether or not you agreed with Frankel, the whole question of patient fees was a "burning idea."[95]

Clearly, much had changed for both the visiting nurse and the VNAs. Like most voluntary medical organizations, their numbers had expanded and their organizations had become more complex. As they grew, so did their annual budgets, and not surprisingly, they attempted to extend their domain beyond the sick poor to encompass patients who could pay for their care. Simultaneously, a variety of measures was implanted to help contain growing budgets by increasing organizational efficiency.

Although for a time lady managers dominated policy in these matters, they inevitably found that their growing enterprises required more attention and expertise than they could provide. While continuing their fundraising and other supportive activities, the ladies were forced to turn to the nurses to reorganize and manage the organizations they had created.

Chapter 3

The Hope and Promise of Public Health

By the end of the nineteenth century, "conservation" was becoming a major concern of social critics. For those who advocated planned use and scientific management of natural resources and national wealth, it was clear that health was a basic resource. Conservation of human resources was essential if the country was to have the large, productive workforce it required.[1]

Believing it was possible to protect the population from both infectious and many noninfectious diseases, a heterogeneous group of public and voluntary organizations emerged during the first two decades of the twentieth century, each accepting responsibility for various aspects of the campaign.[2] Nationally, these efforts were promoted through the establishment of organizations such as the National Association for the Study and Prevention of Tuberculosis in 1905, the American Association for the Study of Prevention of Infant Mortality in 1909, and the Federal Children's Bureau in 1912 and later through the passage of the Sheppard-Towner Act in 1921.

Locally, efforts proceeded in a similar categorical and chaotic fashion with numerous organizations promoting a wide variety of preventive programs. Paralleling and often indistinguishable from these activities were those associated with the Americanization movement. Personal habits, customs, hygiene, and standards of household life, while of immediate concern to those hoping to transform new immigrants into Americans, were at the same time clearly matters of health. It took another thirty years to untangle and coordinate these divergent yet often overlapping activities. What institution should be used or created to provide which services under what circumstances and how much responsibility would be assumed by government, individual, or voluntary organizations were questions yet unanswered.[3]

For the visiting nurse, these circumstances created a time of unlimited possibilities. Already well established in the homes of the poor, she was the logical choice, as one medical authority suggested, to serve as "the relay station, to carry the power from the control stations of science, the hospital, and the university to the individual homes of the community."[4] She would teach individuals how to reduce their susceptibility to disease through alterations in daily habits. Through her lessons on good personal and moral hygiene, fresh air, sunshine, cleanliness, exercise, proper clothing, and diet, health would be restored and disease prevented.[5]

Adelaide Nutting was prophetic when she suggested in 1910 that it was doubtful that many nurses fully grasped the real significance of the situation. In what she called "health nursing," there seemed "to be opening up . . . a field of truly enormous importance, in which the work to be done was large in its scope, attractive in its variety and, to the thoughtful worker, more interesting, because more constructive than that of nursing the sick."[6] This was hardly nursing in the ordinary sense of the term.

Although they were the creation of the visiting nurse association (VNA) the responsibility for these preventive programs was rapidly given over to local boards of health and education. An inevitable, though seemingly unexpected, consequence was the limitation of the activities of these publicly supported nurses to the prevention of disease, leaving the care of the sick to the VNAs. Consequently, while this "new public health" movement provided nursing an opportunity for professional autonomy, status, and employment, it did so in an arena beyond the reach of the nursing leadership who steadfastly retained their allegiance to the VNA.[7]

I

By 1910, death rates, especially for infectious diseases, were declining, and public health officials showed no hesitation in claiming their share of the success. It was through what one author termed "public hygiene" that these diseases had been successfully combated: care of the water supply, food supply, and milk supply; removal of garbage, ashes, and dirt; the cleaning of streets; disposal of sewage; better housing; and the control of contagious disease.[8] But freedom from disease no longer depended simply on community effort or the construction of more public works. There was nothing to be gained by uplifting the masses, it was argued, unless each individual in the mass was to lift himself, for "the effort of the few in trying to change the exterior conditions of the many is love labor lost."[9] Winning the fight against disease now required taking the next step from public hygiene to personal hygiene. This campaign would focus on the affairs of the household and the conduct of the individual's life: "What happens to the bottle of milk after delivery? How are the dishes washed in the kitchen sink? Who uses another person's towel in the common bath?" These were the questions of greatest importance.[10]

If public health was indeed an increasingly private matter, the task ahead required translating the knowledge of scientific medicine into terms of personal effort and responsibility. Education, declared C.-E. A. Winslow, a leading proponent of this view, was the keynote of the modern campaign for public health. The task was enormous, since the ignorance of average Americans concerning the preservation of their health was vast.[11]

For those individuals above the poverty line whose "habits and circumstances of living," it was believed, protected them as a rule from disease, mass methods, exhibits, lectures, and the press seemed sufficient.[12] Education of the poor was by far the more difficult undertaking. The "new idea" of this campaign was to bring "hygienic knowledge right to the individual in his home or shop." This approach would prove more successful with the poor, since the information taught could be adapted to the particular circumstances of each individual and presented in the words of the kitchen, the sitting room, or the boys' club.[13]

In actuality, this idea of a health visitor originated with Florence Nightingale and was first discussed in this country in 1893 at the International Congress of Charities, Correction and Philanthropy.[14] In her widely read paper "Sick Nursing and Health Nursing" and a subsequent paper on "Health Teaching in Towns and Villages," she outlined the details of this new scheme, which she had helped initiate in 1892.[15] In the Nightingale plan, these health missionaries were to be ladies with special training and practical instruction, not district nurses whose work would remain the care of the sick.[16] By 1918, the number of health visitors employed by local communities in England had grown to 3,038.[17]

The only significant variation in the American version of the Nightingale plan was the substitution of the visiting nurse for the lady health missionaries as the teachers of positive health.[18] The nurse was "pre-eminently fitted," explained Winslow, for this function because she was a woman and therefore possessed the patience and tact necessary to bring hygiene into the life of the tenements. Unlike the social worker, she knew the human body and what he described as its reaction to external conditions and to the hygienic conduct of life. Her approach was far superior to that of the physician because she was trained to see the body as a whole, while the physician's vision was distorted by a preoccupation with special pathological conditions.[19] Most nurses shared this viewpoint, adding that most doctors merely diagnosed disease, finding neither the time nor the opportunity to teach health.[20]

Some believed this new field of health nursing differed so greatly from sick nursing that it might, one day, constitute a distinct profession.[21] The nurse entering this field was establishing a unique area of practice, one in which her increased autonomy from the medical profession was expected to create unprecedented opportunity. Her "great and undisputed province" would lie in "the primitive, educational need of protection for a healthy human race."[22] Why not, queried one editorial in the *Public Health Nurse* (*PHN*), "come boldly forth, one and all, and claim the right to exercise the promotion of health as a profession?" After all, the best-educated nurses spent as many years in training to exercise their profession as did the physician to prepare for the "care and scientific prevention of disease."[23] Asserting the obvious independence of their profession, those nurses declared an end to "the old teaching" of the nurse as the handmaiden of the physician. She was instead an associate or coworker of the physician who helped him produce results he could never accomplish alone. Some physicians might still expect to find the nurse waiting "at his elbow," but other, more progressive physicians would surely choose to give nursing "a helping hand" by strengthening her new position.[24]

While home nursing was much less under the control of the physician than hospital nursing, in the case of health nursing, this was particularly true. Although these nurses still carried out the doctor's orders, their new working conditions made it possible to discriminate as to doctors, cooperating with those working for "a higher standard of public welfare" while standing in but "remote and casual relation with those who have no such aims or desire." Even more intimidating to some physicians was the nurse's easy access to the homes of potential patients. For while never diagnosing, these nurses did believe it their business to select those cases requiring diagnosis, sending them where this might best be accomplished.[25]

In the care of the tuberculosis patient, for example, the nurse was, according to Ellen LaMotte, an early leader in the field, "singularly independent." There were no special orders; the doctor knew what should be done, and the nurse knew what to do. Further words were, she claimed, unnecessary. Patients could go for months without seeing the doctor or even change physicians, and it would have no significant impact on their care. It was the nurse who was in charge of the patient's care, who was there through the long months of illness, and who moved with the patient from doctor to doctor. Some exploitative or

ignorant physicians reacted to such behavior on the part of nurses with antagonism and opposition, but according to LaMotte, they were simply "holdovers
from a passing regime." In such cases, the nurse simply proceeded with her
duty even if seemingly at cross purposes with the physician.[26]

The scientific basis of the nurse's work was her knowledge of the nature of
disease, that "complex expression of the sum total of the interaction of parasite
and host, a matter of relationship and relativity of many factors."[27] Her focus
was not germs or even the cure of disease but its predisposing causes. To see
the problem otherwise was placing the cart before the horse, as supporters of
this view claimed.[28] The predisposing causes of disease were those things that
lowered vitality or diminished physiological resistance: bad ventilation, poor
and insufficient food or an "ill-balanced" diet, exposure to heat and cold, insufficient exercise, an improper amount of sleep, not enough or too much clothing, contaminated water or milk, and bad habits with regard to stimulants and
other excesses.[29] The understanding of this seemingly complex balance was to
be found in the "laws of modern hygiene," which interestingly were not unlike
the sanitary ideals articulated by Nightingale (with slight modifications made
necessary by the germ theory of disease).[30]

The major doctrines of modern hygiene were sunshine, cleanliness, fresh
air, and pure food.[31] Sunshine was particularly useful, since recent studies had
seemingly demonstrated its ability to kill certain bacteria. It followed that dark
rooms, shaded rooms, or north rooms, while not the cause of disease, were
"distinctly unhealthful and would depress both mental and vital activities,"
leaving an individual defenseless against disease. This law became exceedingly
clear if one simply observed the disastrous effect caused by placing a healthy
plant in the cellar for a few days.[32] Light also provided a secondary benefit in
encouraging cleanliness by "pitilessly" illuminating dust and other materials
"inimical" to good health. Cleanliness was believed to be the best safeguard
against disease. The elimination of dirt, dust, and flies, all carriers of disease,
was the first condition of health, but cleanliness also included people, food,
milk, and water.[33]

Clean, pure air was also essential to good health because it contained life-
giving oxygen. Every hour a man "spoils for further use in breathing" as much
air as contained in a room sixteen by twelve by ten feet. A proper system of
ventilation was essential for good health, for rebreathing expired air with all
its impurities would eventually undercut an individual's health.[34] Impure air
was as harmful to the lungs and general health as tainted meat and spoiled fruit
were unwholesome and bad for the stomach.[35] The teachings of Nightingale
remained in force; windows were made to open in such a fashion to flush the

room with fresh air without causing a draft, while doors and transoms were closed to keep used air from contaminating the rest of the house.[36] Finally, a proper diet was essential. To ensure good health, cheap and indigestible foods, such as cabbage, turnips, doughnuts, and pies, must be replaced by nourishing food, such as fish, meat, eggs, rice, beans, hominy, and oatmeal.[37]

While believing that health in the home would ultimately mean health everywhere, spokesmen for the visiting nurse also emphasized that the chain of health was only as strong as its weakest link.[38] The acceptance of such views would no doubt have created an endless set of responsibilities for the health nurse. Her first task was to enter the homes of the poor as a "scientific investigator" whose aim was to study the moral as well as physical conditions of the whole family, "to root out the causes of illness."[39] Having diagnosed a home's problems, the nurse's next responsibility was to show its inhabitants the way to health. The successful nurse had the ability to "impress her points upon others and to make them see that what she proposes is right, reasonable and advantageous."[40] Often it was not enough to simply tell the family; frequently, they had to be shown. Patience was an "essential part of the nurse's equipment," for she "must be willing to reiterate over and over again without showing annoyance, the rules which have been needlessly and exasperatingly ignored." No one knows better than the nurse, declared LaMotte, "the awful hiatus that exists between preaching and practicing—the glib promise and the broken pledge."[41]

While acknowledging the opportunities created by this new area of endeavor, several leading nurses questioned whether the lives and homes of the poor provided the proper opportunity for successfully teaching the laws of hygiene.[42] For the domain of the poor was, as Mrs. Isabel Lowman graphically described it, at the end of a very narrow, dark alley where garbage and refuse covered the steps and ground with a kind of "loathsome litter" and where the floor was covered with banana peels, sticks, straws, dirt, and bits of food. Where, as if the disorder was not discouraging enough, the "slatternly neighborhood woman" was weaving endlessly, wandering "back and forth and around the dirty kitchen."[43]

Opportunity was, as Charlotte Aiken pointed out to her audience at the 1906 National Conference of Charities and Corrections, "the suitable combination of conditions for executing a purpose." "What can you hope to teach when you find these conditions?" she queried. What permanent results should be expected?[44] What use is it to insist that a pregnant woman should have plenty of nourishing food when "the whole family lives on baker's bread and a few green vegetables" cooked in oil or to talk of cleanliness when a family of eight occupies one room and takes in boarders?[45] She concluded that where the conditions "that make for cleanliness and virtue and self-respect are wanting," there could be no real opportunity for educational work. Palliative advice could be given, sickness made less dreadful, and a little comfort provided, but anything more, she suggested, was "useless tinkering."[46]

After several years of working with tuberculosis patients, LaMotte was reluctantly forced to share these views. Ten years before, when she first entered the field, she naively believed tuberculosis was both preventable and curable. Simple education about the nature of disease and its transmissibility and spread was all that was needed to produce good results. Unfortunately, she found her theory was nearly impossible to put into practice because her patients were poor and thus lacked willpower, intelligence, and self-control. For the same reason, their environment was difficult to alter and cure almost impossible to obtain.[47] Eventually, she was forced to conclude that the nurses' teachings, no matter how thorough and conscientious, were simply halfway measures; at best, she could hope to produce only momentary cooperation.[48]

Most of these critics agreed with Mary Lent, superintendent of the Baltimore Visiting Nurses, that the failure of education as a method of suppressing disease was due to the fact that even with all the help they received, the poor were unable to apply consistently and unflaggingly what they learned to their daily lives. Families below the poverty line simply did not have the means for carrying out the principles of hygiene, nor did their surroundings permit it.[49] Those who had been in the field the longest and were now willing to admit the truth agreed, Lent declared, that at best,

> we are but Red Cross nurses in the field of battle. For years we have been giving temporary relief in the way of skilled nursing care, under conditions that deprive it of three-quarters of its value. We have also been trying to teach underpaid, overworked, underfed, wretched human beings how to live more hygienic lives. But the awakening has come at last. Our eyes are now open to the facts. We can no longer continue to dole out surface relief and believe that it stands for anything more radical. It is for us, who are palliative agents, to declare that the conditions of today do not call for palliative treatment.[50]

She concluded that the nurse's most valuable work was the collection of facts about the conditions that demanded nursing care while simultaneously defeating nursing's efforts. It was the duty of the public health nurse to present these facts to the public "in such an array and in such numbers that they can neither be contradicted nor ignored."[51] Many other visiting nurses shared Lent's view that the problems of the poor required social reform more than hygienic instruction. Wald went so far as to suggest that impressing upon the poor the last word of science without simultaneously urging reform in housing, child protection, and wages was "cruelly sardonic on the part of the nurse."[52]

II

Despite such reservations, visiting nursing willingly embarked on this new educational venture. By 1910, the majority of the large urban VNAs had initiated new preventive programs for schoolchildren, infants, mothers, and patients with tuberculosis. Not only was the focus of these programs a radical departure from tradition, but the methods used by the lady managers to finance them were equally unprecedented. Unable to finance any large new programs, the ladies used two methods to entice others to pay for these new works—the joint venture and the demonstration. In the joint venture, the VNA provided the nurses and some other voluntary organization provided the money. Demonstrations were a bit more risky, since in those instances, the VNA initiated the program on a small-scale, experimental basis, assuming that when its worth was clear to "the public," the necessary funds would be provided.

School nursing best illustrates the demonstration approach to expansion. In many cities, physicians had been hired by the city to inspect schoolchildren and to exclude those with contagious diseases. Initially, this approach presented few problems, but as the number of children excluded grew rapidly, many boards of education began to seek other solutions. By 1902, the situation in New York City schools was out of control, with fifteen to twenty children per school being sent home daily. At the suggestion of Wald, a nurse from the Henry Street Settlement House was sent to four schools to demonstrate how, through the home visits of a nurse, the illnesses of these children could be cured. The experiment was successful, and at the end of a month, the board of health hired twelve nurses and appropriated $30,000 to continue this work. The efficiency of the program was further documented by a dramatic decrease in absenteeism from 63,175 children in 1903 to 5,455 in 1909. By 1910, the staff had increased to 140 nurses.[53]

In Boston, this work was launched in 1906 with two nurses, one supported by the Instructive District Nurse Association (IDNA) and the other by the members of the Fathers and Mothers Club. Later that year, five more IDNA nurses were added. As in New York City, the work began as an experiment, "knowing that if it was successful . . . it would be only a question of time when the public would see its importance and come to their support." But unlike New York City, it took a bit longer than anticipated for the city to take up this program.[54] A bill introduced by the Massachusetts Civic League was finally passed by the legislature in 1907, appropriating sufficient funds for twenty nurses.

The superintendent of schools hoped the district nurses would take the school nurse exam "as they are doing such a good job," but none cared to work for the city.[55]

In Philadelphia, the Visiting Nurse Society (VNS) had to resort to more dramatic tactics before funds were appropriated for a school nurse program. In 1903, Dr. Martin, director of Public Charities, made available the money to pay a VNS nurse to assist with medical inspection in the schools. The same year, the Public Education Association of Philadelphia, with the cooperation of the VNS petitioned the city council, requesting that $1,800 be appropriated for the salaries for two school nurses.[56] Nothing happened, and by 1906, the lady managers were forced to conclude that there was "very little prospect of the appointment of a staff of nurses for the schools in the near future."[57] In June 1907, they decided to force the issue by "enlarging the experiment and giving it more publicity." An appeal was sent to the principals and inspecting physicians inquiring whether they would like six additional school nurses. The nurses were placed in the schools in October, and in November, the board of education was notified that the VNS would only pay the nurses' salaries until January. Thus forced to act, the board of education somehow acquired sufficient funds for one supervisor and five school nurses. The VNS was victorious at last.[58]

VNAs also assumed an important role in the campaign against tuberculosis. By the turn of the century, it had become clear that although medical science was now able to provide a great deal of information about tuberculosis and specific guidance as to its prevention, no prompt or simple medical solution was forthcoming. The campaign would require many more clinics and sanatoriums, but more importantly, any progress required the overcoming of public apathy and ignorance.[59]

Tuberculosis was seen as a "house disease" of the very poor, and its elimination required the personal cooperation of patients and their families. Since tuberculosis caused about 10 percent of all deaths and as much as 15 percent in some cities its eradication required the cooperation of thousands of families.[60]

The visiting nurse seemed ideally suited for this task, and not surprisingly, VNAs were among the first voluntary societies working to combat tuberculosis. But many, like the Philadelphia society, quickly found that this was their most expensive program, since the patients tended to be poverty-stricken and often required time-consuming teaching before the nurse was able to bring about the total reordering of the household thought necessary. Recognizing the magnitude of this undertaking, visiting nurse societies were careful, as one Boston lady manager put it, to avoid allowing anyone to place responsibility for the

whole tuberculosis movement with their organization. The glory of the VNA
would come from initiating the work, not in bearing its long-term financial burden. Financing this educational campaign was, in their view, the responsibility
of the growing number of voluntary societies for the prevention of tuberculosis
and, ultimately, the city government.[61]

Thus the role of VNAs in the development of the campaign against tuberculosis was most frequently that of partners in a joint venture. Typical of
this approach was the work initiated by Dr. and Mrs. Lowman in Cleveland.
Dr. Lowman was a member of the Western Reserve Medical School faculty,
and Mrs. Lowman was an active member of the board of the Cleveland VNA.
Both were concerned about the lack of services for tuberculosis patients, and
in 1903, they went to Germany and France to study the treatment of con-
sumption abroad. Following their trip, Dr. Lowman began to open tuberculosis dispensaries—four by 1905—while Mrs. Lowman and her committee on
tuberculosis began to raise money to provide VNA staff visits to the dispensary patients. With the help of the Lowmans, the Cleveland Anti-Tuberculosis
League was organized in 1905, and by 1908, it was able to assume all expenses
for the tuberculosis nurses. In September 1910, the league presented a report
on tuberculosis conditions in the city to the mayor, and as a result, the Bureau
of Tuberculosis was established in the department of health. By 1913, all tuberculosis nursing was being financed by the city, which saw itself, as one health
officer suggested, as having "come to the rescue and provided funds for the
support of the work."[62]

As the campaign grew, many organizations began to follow the lead of
VNAs and hired nurses to visit their tuberculosis patients at home. By 1914,
there were four thousand visiting nurses doing the tuberculosis work for dispensaries, hospital outpatient departments, health departments, VNAs, and
voluntary tuberculosis societies.[63] But in cities like New York, where forty-nine
different organizations were sending tuberculosis nurses into the community,
duplication and confusion were inevitable. Despite efforts to avoid these problems, many cities were never able to establish efficient, cooperative relationships among the various organizations.[64]

Paralleling this growth in the number and variety of organizations caring for tuberculosis patients was a steady increase in government support for
those programs at the state and municipal levels. This was especially true in
more progressive states like New York and Pennsylvania, where by 1910, the
proportion of government to total expenditures was 60 percent and 70 percent,
respectively. According to Richard Shryock, by 1910, public appropriation for
tuberculosis work nationally was more than $9 million annually. The VNAs

actively supported this trend, as did many voluntary tuberculosis societies, since the outcome was often programs far beyond their individual financial capabilities.[65]

The New York City Health Department had one of the most impressive tuberculosis programs during this period, with a $250,000 budget and a staff of 159 visiting nurses in 1910.[66] At the same time, in Baltimore, Cleveland, Philadelphia, and Boston, either city or state departments of health had begun to accept major responsibility for tuberculosis work. The VNAs continued to care for the bedridden tuberculosis patient, while the city nurses' primary responsibilities were educational and preventive.[67] In Philadelphia, for example, the VNS cared for an average of two hundred to three hundred tuberculosis patients per year, while the Boston nurses visited about four hundred each year. In some cities, like Detroit and Chicago, the visiting nurses associations continued to do most of the work with tuberculosis patients, with the local tuberculosis society financing at least half of the cost of the program.[68]

Like tuberculosis, infant welfare programs began in many cities as a cooperative venture between several voluntary societies and, eventually, the city. Infant mortality—the number of babies dying before one year of age—had become for most industrialized nations the symbolic indicator of national health status. By their "quick and dirty" criteria, turn-of-the-century America, with approximately 1 out of every 7 infants dying, was indeed in poor health. The children of foreign-born parents experienced the highest mortality, with 149 babies dying out of every 1,000 births. This was in contrast to the 135 deaths per 1,000 births for children of native-born parents.[69]

As in many turn-of-the-century campaigns to prevent or control disease, the immigrant became the main focus of infant welfare work. The maternal and infant welfare conference, milk stations, lessons in infant feeding, and home visits by infant welfare nurses were all elements in this campaign whose major concern was reducing deaths caused by summer diarrhea.[70] Believing that at least 50 percent, and possibly all, of these deaths, were caused by dirty milk, improper feeding, and unhygienic environments, they saw instructing the mother—"reducing her ignorance"—as well as providing clean milk as their goals.[71]

In addition, the campaign to improve child health was, as George Rosen has argued, in part an element in the Americanization movement, an activity that served to assimilate immigrant families. Infant mortality was a practical problem affecting many immigrants, and providing clean milk created the desired opportunity to teach the American way to mothers and, through her, to the family.[72]

Like the campaign against tuberculosis, this program required teachers. Someone was needed to instruct the mothers when they came to have their babies examined or to obtain milk. Someone was also needed to visit the home to investigate the living conditions and make any necessary modifications in the patient's environment. Thus the visiting nurse came to specialize in infant welfare work. But according to the Philadelphia lady managers, "trying to teach an ignorant mother how to care for her baby is no easy task, especially when she has had several others, and seems to think she knows all there is to know concerning such a small thing, but the nurses never forgot that patience was the keynote to it all and the results were more . . . even than had been hoped for."[73]

There was, according to Mary Gardner, a great demand for maternal education, but as with many new programs, financial support was limited. Money was needed for other programs, and more significantly, many viewed infant welfare as a municipal responsibility.[74] The New York City Health Department was the first to establish such a program in 1903 when it began sending school nurses to visit sick infants during summer months. In 1908, the city established the Division of Child Hygiene and eventually assumed major responsibility for infant welfare.[75]

In Philadelphia, infant welfare work was begun in 1906 as a cooperative effort of the Starr Center and the VNS. In 1908, the Starr Center, which was a voluntary association whose primary concern was babies, took over the work, hiring its own nurses. A child hygiene division was established by the city in 1910, and with the help of the VNS, nurses conducted a door-to-door survey in search of all infants needing care. By 1916, Philadelphia had a staff of sixty nurses doing this work. Unlike most city nurses, they cared for all children, sick and well.[76]

Cleveland had a similar experience with the VNS and the infant clinics of the Milk Fund, initiating this work in 1906 and later transferring it to the city.[77] Infant welfare work in Boston was started by the Baby Hygiene Association, which was taken over by the IDNA in 1922 only to find itself in such financial difficulties that by 1924, a large part of the well-baby and preschool work had to be transferred to the health department.[78]

But the concerns of the visiting nurse were never confined simply to the infant, for even prior to the turn of the century, many large VNAs provided care for mothers as well, although these early obstetrical programs were limited to postpartum care. By 1900, many associations began to extend these programs to include the prenatal period, believing that infant and maternal mortality could be reduced more rapidly if the mother's health was supervised throughout her pregnancy.[79] But visiting nurses found little support for their views. The health reformers had not, as yet, recognized maternal mortality as a public health problem, and the medical profession was still busy debating what constituted good obstetrical care. As Antler and Fox demonstrated, it was not until the 1920s and the passage of the Sheppard-Towner Act that the movement toward a safe maternity was actually initiated. This legislation, largely the work of a national women's lobby, provided federal grants to states and made it possible for thousands of prenatal and infant care programs to be started.[80]

But in the meantime, undaunted by lack of public support, VNAs had taken on prenatal care as an important aspect of their work. Over the years, this program continued to grow until it came to constitute 25–30 percent of the services provided.[81] By the time prenatal care was taken up as a favorite strategy by health reformers, VNAs had lost any inclination toward relinquishing their maternity programs. Thus because of its distinctive development dynamics, prenatal care evolved in a fashion quite different from the preventive programs for tuberculosis; schoolchildren and infants were initiated by VNAs with the full intent of transferring them to the city at the first opportunity. Increasingly, the work of the VNAs would be confined to the care of sick and pregnant women, while boards of health and education would assume major responsibility for preventive services generally.[82]

Clearly, much had changed for both the visiting nurse and VNAs during this period. Having emerged from what Gardner called their pioneer stage, visiting nurses were enjoying a time of both hope and promise.[83] Not surprisingly, the number of agencies seeking their services had increased from only 115 in 1900 to nearly 2,000 by 1914. Visiting nurses could be found working for department stores, factories, insurance companies, boards of health and education, hospitals, settlement houses, milk and baby clinics, playgrounds, and hotels, as well as for VNAs. Visiting nursing held the promise of becoming an important new field of employment for nurses, which would enhance the overall reputation of the nursing profession while ensuring its autonomy and public support.[84]

Similarly, the lady managers were enjoying a great deal of success, having launched numerous new programs of clear importance to the public's health.[85] But what at the turn of the century had been a manageable philanthropic activity for ladies of leisure was expanding into a major enterprise that often demanded more than they could provide. While the ladies proceeded as best they could, the consequences of their judgment remain at issue today.[86]

The outcome of this rapid growth in preventive services varied from city to city, with voluntary and official agencies assuming essentially unpredictable, often overlapping, responsibilities.[87] As the confusion grew, so did the debate as to the relative functions of the voluntary (or, as they were often called, "non-official") and the official health agencies. The central concern was, of course, one of control.[88]

Voluntary organizations saw themselves as fulfilling a set of responsibilities that they could accomplish with "peculiar fitness and effectiveness." Their great advantage was that they were managed by men and women who were "mobile, curious and, to a certain extent, independent in the exercise of their ability and unhampered by unfriendly criticism."[89] Claiming to have come into existence because of the imperfections of the official health agencies, they saw their purpose as assisting or supplementing official activities through education, research, demonstration, and standardization. Health officers, they argued, could not attend to the "myriad details of their administrative work and conduct investigations or research." Nor could the health department be justified in using taxpayers' money to test new methods of work. It was, therefore, the task of the voluntary agency to conduct this experimental program. Once the work of a particular program was established, public interest was aroused, and the most effective methods were established, the official agency could, they argued, easily obtain expansion funds as a part of a governmental program.

Thus voluntary agencies saw themselves as a cornerstone of public health work and, as Mrs. Lowman described it, "an experimental laboratory whose cost in energy and money must ever be a surtax on the good will of the private individual." While admitting that at some point all health activities might conceivably be taken over by public departments, the voluntary agencies claimed that the time had not yet come. Organizations for community health were far from complete, and health officers were far from wise and content with limited progress, while the public was not educated to the point of recognizing the need to provide sufficient money for health programs.[90]

In contrast, some health officers tended not to see the activities of voluntary health organizations as supportive or cooperative but as competitive and self-serving. They saw the activities of voluntary organizations as misplaced; instead of directing their efforts toward strengthening the official agencies, they chose instead to create new organizations and programs.[91] The growing popularity of public health, declared Dr. Frances Curtis (chairman of the Newton, Massachusetts, Board of Health), causes clever people to see it as a means for justifying the existence of their nonofficial agencies: "They apparently wish to appropriate all the successes which the pioneers of public health have achieved, use them for their own advantages, and leave for the Board of Health only such parts of the work as they themselves cannot do because of lack of legal authority."[92]

Another physician, Carl McCombs of the New York Bureau of Municipal Research, claimed that studies had clearly shown that the failure of many health officers to perform effectively was due in large measure to this divided responsibility. Bound by no limitations except funds and responsible to no one but their financial supporters, the private health agencies had grown so rapidly that McCombs claimed the health officer was beginning to wonder "whether he was the ringmaster or only the clown in the circus."[93]

According to both physicians, private health organizations had "mistaken their functions and misunderstood their relationship to government." Private organizations needed to be put in their proper place: "standing back of and helping the official agencies, placing themselves at the disposal of the health officer and permitting him to direct their activities according to his plan."[94] There was hardly a function of public health that the board of health could not perform better than the nonofficial agencies, they claimed. If, instead of trying to strengthen their own organizations and their own grip upon the public health programs, private agencies studied the needs of the health departments, assisting in their fight for larger appropriations, better and more permanent health benefits would have resulted.[95]

Such contradictory views must account to some degree for the overlapping and confusing health-care systems that evolved over the years in many major cities. For, as Haven Emerson (at one time a health officer in New York City), later remembered, "competition and rivalry in methods, resources, and accomplishments became as keen as in selling soap or advertising toothpaste."[96]

III

Nurses entering this new profession experienced, according to Dock, a practical compulsion toward specialization—limiting their work to one age group or disease. Infants, tuberculosis, pregnant women, and schoolchildren had all become objects of incipient specialization.[97] Some argued that for nursing to achieve the "highest possibilities" in these new endeavors, it was necessary to devote all their time to a particular area and "by so doing become experts in it, able to lead others, able to contribute to the literature. . . . In short, to do for the nursing profession what the specialist in medicine [was] so successfully doing for the medical profession."[98] Being a specialist appealed to nurses. It seemed scientific, progressive, and "efficient."[99] Possibly even more important was the reality that nurses who specialized found themselves in demand and in line for promotion in their particular field, while those who did not, as one nurse suggested, went "around and around in a circle" and were no more on the way to advancement at the end of the year than at its beginning.[100]

In actuality, nurses who specialized in these new preventive roles found it difficult to combine their educational functions with caring for the "bodily needs" of patients. To many, it seemed unreasonable to think that nurses would take time for health teaching while their sick patients were waiting for a bath or treatment, and increasingly, the roles diverged.[101] Nurses themselves rarely objected to this new division of labor, for health nursing certainly left them less physically and mentally tired at the end of each day. By distancing herself from the bedside, she was, in addition, elevating herself to the superior status of thinker.[102] She was more than a nurse—more than, as one supporter of this view suggested, "a parasitic profession fattening upon the disease of humanity." No longer "the white linen nurse . . . beautiful, and clean, fair skinned and timid eyed," she had become "the red-blooded nurse with force, power and determination."[103] Given all the advantages of this new work, women of education would at last be attracted to nursing, and that alone would be desirable for the profession.[104]

As boards of health and education rapidly came to be the major employers of these nurses, elimination of bedside care increasingly became the rule. Despite much ongoing debate as to the appropriate domain of public health practice, the focus of health departments became increasingly preventive. Most health officers willingly abandoned claims to any curative activities that might be construed as threatening the economic well-being of private physicians.[105] What they chose for themselves, they not surprisingly chose for their employees, and accordingly, many health officers believed the work of the public health nurse was hygienic, not therapeutic. Nurses who spent any significant amount of their time providing bedside care should not in the estimation of such public health leaders be classified as public health nurses.[106]

The nursing leadership, many of them superintendents of VNAs, were outraged by such assertions.[107] Visiting nurses, they insisted, had always been teachers of prevention and hygiene and had in fact "blazed the trail" for all these new specialized groups. The visiting nurse, unlike most specialists, had had the wisdom to see the value of caring for the sick as a means of gaining access to families in greatest need of health education. Because she cared for the sick, the visiting nurse was more effectively able to "permanently better the conditions" of those families under her care. Nurses who were simply teachers could have no such impact on the family. Were health officers' assertions that visiting nurses were not public health nurses made, they wondered, "to keep the visiting nurse in her place, outside the sphere of public health work?" If so, their efforts were in vain for, proclaimed their leaders, the visiting nurse was as much a public health nurse as any nurse employed by the health departments.[108]

Visiting nurses who envisioned themselves as general practitioners, ministering to all the needs of their community, assumed an increasingly antagonistic attitude toward specialization. Because public health nurses were so specialized and unwilling to care for the sick, they were causing significant problems for the community, the nurse, and families.[109] The result, claimed most prominent visiting nurses, was duplication in transportation, supervision, and overhead. Even worse was the duplication that occurred in the home when one family could potentially be visited by the baby nurse, the tuberculosis nurse, the maternity nurse, the contagion nurse, the school nurse, and the visiting nurse. Even with this great amount of people going into the home advising and educating, Wald mused ironically, it was possible that the patient might not be bathed or have his wound dressed. For most patients, this situation seemed hopeless, as no group of agencies was capable of sustaining the level of cooperation required to eliminate such chaos.[110]

For the nurse who specialized, the critics predicted an equally disastrous outcome. She, they suggested, would eventually become a depressed victim of sterile routine. Even worse, she would be faced too often with the tragic situation of having to refuse "real care" to her patients at a time of illness.[111] The greatest mistake made by visiting nursing was to separate the care of the sick from the teaching of prevention; the solution was simply to put them back together. The public health nurse must again become what Winslow called the "community mother," the trained and scientific representative of the good neighbor, caring for all—sick and well.[112]

While they argued their case at conventions and in the journals, at home, the visiting nurses found they had little control outside their own organizations.[113] Ironically, while they had created a pattern of service delivery that would shape the future of public health nursing for years to come, they found the outcome less than welcome.[114]

Chapter 4

Preserving the Treasures of Their Tradition

The Founding of the National Organization for Public Health Nursing and the Red Cross Rural Nursing Service

The year 1912 was triumphal for visiting nurses who, declared Lillian Wald, were finally in the position they had dreamed of for years. At last, they had the opportunity to promote and actually establish visiting nurse services nationwide.[1] The reasons for Wald's enthusiasm were the newly created Red Cross Rural Nursing Service and the National Organization for Public Health Nursing (NOPHN). What the Rural Nursing Service would do for those in the country, the Nation Organization for Public Health Nursing would do for city dwellers. Not only would the services of the visiting nurse become available nationwide, but they would also develop under the careful control and protection of the visiting nurse leadership.

Despite the appearance of having made significant gains in professional control, both organizations relied heavily on financial assistance provided by a few wealthy laymen and women. This dependence on private benevolence was a long-standing tradition, and as long as the nurses were allowed to exercise the authority of their newfound status, little tension existed between them and their lay supporters.

The entrance of the United States into World War I turned harmony and cooperation into competition for control. In their efforts to keep pace with both the demands as well as the opportunities created by the war, the two organizations frequently found themselves pursuing radically different, often conflicting, solutions. By the end of the war, the NOPHN, despite its apparent achievements, found itself constantly confronted by what appeared to be the expansionist tendencies of the Red Cross.

The demands of war also accelerated the NOPHN's financial dependence on its lay supporters and ultimately brought to an end nursing's uncontested domination of the organization. Tired of paying the bills while having no control, Frances Payne Bolton was the first to campaign for equal status for lay contributors on the board of directors. The nurses had two choices: either antagonize Bolton or incur the wrath of the profession by violating nursing's "closed door" policy. The nurses chose to acquiesce to Bolton's request. This chapter examines the developments within and between the NOPHN and the Red Cross Rural Nursing Service from their inception through the end of World War I.

I

Visiting nursing's rapid, even hectic and confusing, growth brought more services to the poor and led to the development of an important new field of employment for nurses. But it also created what would become an increasingly severe problem. Evolving agency by agency, visiting nursing grew up outside of the control of the nursing profession. Of major concern to the visiting nurse leadership was the proliferation of small agencies whose boards of directors were, they believed, neophytes acting out of total ignorance—unaware of the answers to the most elementary questions. How else, they queried, could their failure to seek the advice of the nurses in charge of the older, well-established organizations be explained? Obviously, declared Mary Gardner, they were simply blundering along, "doing not only harm to their own community, but retarding the advance of the whole movement."[2] Although leading visiting nurses saw danger in this situation, they did not act promptly or in a sufficiently organized fashion to systemically influence what was developing.[3]

The vulnerable situation of visiting nursing began to be seriously discussed by the movement's leadership in 1911. As one member of the board of the Cleveland Visiting Nurse Association (VNA) observed at the time, "We find quite suddenly that matters of method and of ethics can be left to the mercy of general interpretation only so long as no powerful suggestion to construe them unusually is made from without."[4] Her rather vague words of warning were, in fact, a response to just such a suggestion. Ella Crandall and Wald, both leading public health nurses, had recently learned of a proposal made by Dr. Lee Frankel, vice president of the Metropolitan Life Insurance Company (MLI), to the boards of the Chicago and Boston VNAs. Addressing his request to the two associations that were in the midst of reorganization and without the guidance of a superintendent of nurses, Frankel had asked the boards to add practical nurses to their staffs to take care of chronic patients. By thus hiring less experienced attendants, Frankel hoped to reduce the nursing services that the Metropolitan had agreed to provide to its industrial policyholders during illness. The nursing profession could no longer ignore the influence of "Mother Met."[5]

Responding swiftly to Frankel's plan, leaders of organized nursing discussed the matter privately with Frankel and publicly in nursing journals.[6]
Edna Foley (the superintendent-elect of the Chicago association) wrote, for
example, an article in which the proposal's risks to patients were made clear.
Foley asked rhetorically whether Frankel's request meant that VNAs were
"intended to care for the sick or to act as investigating agents and supervisors for commercial interest." She wondered whether standards had been "so
lowered that only the number of visits and the amounts of instruction given
counts, while the actual work of our hands has become so unimportant that it
can with safety and expedition be handed over to so-called practical nurses,
whose practice is on a par with the scanty remuneration they receive." Finally,
she asserted in conclusion, "the poor are at the mercy of too many half-trained
and counterfeit workers as it is, and it behooves the visiting nurse associations
in good standing to maintain the integrity of our calling by offering their best
alike to the acute and the chronic sick."[7]

Despite their strong stand against the Metropolitan proposal, nurses did
recognize that many chronic patients could get along without expensive expert
care. Nevertheless, since they were still struggling to convince the public that
expert nursing care was important, nurses felt called upon to resist this potential threat to fragile public confidence. At a New York Academy of Medicine
meeting, Annie Goodrich (a leading nurse), described their potion this way: "If
there is another body or class of workers needed, it will come into existence;
we believed, indeed, that such a class is here and is only waiting to come into
an orderly existence for the field of the more important worker, the nurse, to be
developed . . . if the doctor and the family are satisfied to relegate their sick to
her hands, well and good. Our responsibility ceases. Our point had been made
when the line of demarcation is clear."[8]

Obviously, however, no such line of demarcation as the one Goodrich
called for had been made for the visiting nurse. Indeed, Frankel's efforts to
develop a special kind of nursing care for the chronically ill pushed to the
forefront an issue of professional self-definition that visiting nurses were not
yet prepared to resolve.

In the end, Frankel was convinced to drop his plan, although he did succeed in reducing the company's expenditures for the care or chronic patients.
Arguing that service to the acutely ill demonstrated larger practical returns, he
eventually virtually eliminated services to the chronically ill. More important,
however, Frankel's proposal provided the impetus needed to convince visiting
nurses to organize themselves.[9] As Mrs. Isabel Lowman described what many

had learned, organization was now thought necessary if "the treasures of their tradition" were to "be preserved intact."[10]

In January of 1912, Wald became chairwoman of a committee formed by the American Nurses' Association and the America Society of Superintendents of Training Schools to consider the possibility of creating a national VNA.[11] Realizing that nursing's ideals would be protected only if shared by the members of VNA boards, their goal was to formulate an association that by its very nature would ensure this outcome. All that was really required was education; when properly informed, board members would, no doubt, share the nurses' convictions. Many proposals were considered by the committee before they finally concluded that the active participation of board members in this new association would prove the more efficient mode of guaranteeing such needed "education."[12]

In an effort to ensure support for their proposal, the committee wrote to all the 1,092 organizations employing visiting nurses, communicating their concerns about the dangers associated with the rapid growth of this field, conveying their conviction that the time was "ripe" for the formation of a national organization, and inviting each agency to send a representative to the nursing convention to discuss these matters. Of the eighty responses to their inquiry, sixty-nine indicated a willingness to send a delegate to the proposed meeting.[13]

Satisfied that sufficient support existed, the nurses proceeded with their task. As a result of three more meetings, the committee attended the convention armed with not only their recommendations but a "temporary" constitution for the new organization they were confident would emerge from it.[14]

The national nursing convention was held in Chicago in June 1912. Gardner presented the committee's report, and after a day and a half of meetings, the new organization was created.[15] Its objectives were to "stimulate responsibility for the health of the community by the establishing of extensions of visiting nursing and all other forms public health nursing; to facilitate efficient cooperation between nurses, physicians, boards of trustees and other persons interested in public health measures; to develop standards of ethics and techniques of public health nursing services; to establish and maintain a central bureau for information, reference and assistance in matters pertaining to such service and to publish periodicals and issue bulletins from time to time to aid in the general accomplishment of the organization."[16]

The organization's name had been hotly debated. Tradition and sentiment argued for the term *visiting nurse*, but the term was eventually dropped in favor of one thought big enough to cover all the work being done. As Crandall explained it, in the term finally chosen to describe the new organization, the nurses were "borrowing from or banking on the future, rather than the past or present [and] . . . establishing in anticipation a vital connection between visiting nursing and public health."[17]

The NOPHN would be a federation of organizations but would also allow individual membership. "Individual" members were nurses who were graduates of a recognized hospital of no less than fifty beds with a training program lasting at least two years that included obstetrics. These members could participate in all activities and could vote. "Associate" members were nurses who were not eligible for individual membership and individuals who were not nurses—that is, board members. These members were encouraged to participate in all activities but had no vote. Finally, any organization engaged in public health nursing could become a corporate member, and through their nurse delegate, they would have one vote. The fifteen-member board of directors would be elected from among the individual members.[18]

Thus the control of the NOPHN would remain the prerogative of a small group of nurses whose efforts on behalf of visiting nursing would be augmented by the opinions and suggestions of the associate members.[19] Lay women found their standing within the new organization acceptable for the moment. Lay membership, even if nonvoting, was a radical departure from nursing tradition and, at least, symbolically recognized a shared purpose and mutual dependence.

Before the close of the convention, the new organization was presented with two gifts by the lady managers of the VNA of Cleveland. The first was a seal depicting, in a style reminiscent of Maxfield Parrish, a kneeling woman planting a young tree. Its inscription, from Proverbs, reads in full verse: "Hope deferred maketh the heart sick; but when the desire cometh it is a tree of life." It was selected as the NOPHN's national insignia to symbolize the visiting nurse as the restorer of both health and hope.[20]

The second gift offered by the Cleveland board was its publication, the *VNQ*, with its one thousand subscribers, advertising contracts, and remaining budget. Although the official publication of the NOPHN, it became obvious that, at least initially, the *Quarterly*'s management and financial needs would have to remain the responsibility of its Cleveland laywomen founders.[21]

Less well-publicized was the Cleveland ladies' financial sponsorship of the NOPHN, which consistently materialized during periods of financial crisis over the years. An anonymous gift, no doubt from one the Cleveland board members, made it possible for the NOPHN to become the first nursing organization to open an office and hire a full-time executive secretary. Despite this strong bond with Cleveland, the office was open in New York City, and a New Yorker, Crandall, was eventually convinced to give up most of her faculty responsibility at Teachers College to run the organization.[22]

The new organization was formed none too soon. Frankel, concerned that his company's work was seriously hampered by the visiting nurses' "charity image," was about to propose a new scheme. In December of 1912, he approached three of the larger associations, requesting that they separate their staff, keeping one staff for charity work and one to care for MLI's policyholders. The nurses doing "Metropolitan" work would wear a "brevet" and have a separate supervisor who would secretly remain under the control of the VNA. Creating the illusion of a separate nursing organization would, according Frankel, shield policyholders from the appearance of accepting charity.[23]

Hearing of Frankel's latest plot, Crandall, in consultation with the newly formed executive committee of the NOPHN, prepared an article for publication in the next issue of the *Quarterly*. The article concluded that VNAs could not share the motives of the business world, would not become propagandists for commercial concerns, and would prefer "to withdraw from the preset connection with the company than to imperil the spiritual and social implications that are involved in their present relationship to community."[24]

The article was submitted to Frankel in advance, offering him "the privilege of answering in the same issue." Crandall later recounted Frankel's response as that of "indignation and resentment" that the NOPHN was unwilling to at least try out his experiment and judge it on its own merit. Exercising the power of her newly acquired position, Crandall confidently refused, declaring that "if the new organization had any purpose at all, it was warn its constituents in advance instead of later." The disadvantages of Frankel's plan were, in her opinion, "too patent to need experimentation."[25] Frankel finally agreed to postpone his experiment, and in exchange, Crandall's article was never published.

Crandall wrote to the executive committee, admonishing them to remember that although she had negotiated an "amicable adjustment," Frankel's experiment was postponed, not abandoned. She cautioned them to come to the June convention prepared for more negotiations.[26] Mary Beard would later remember these early confrontations with amusement. The nurses actually feared Frankel, she recalled, and it seemed impossible to interpret neither "our professional standards to him nor his profession's needs to us."[27]

Fortunately, the June convention had a catalytic effect on their relationship. Frankel was asked to publicly present his concerns, and his paper "Visiting Nursing from a Business Organization's Standpoint" became the focus of discussion nationwide.[28] By the end of the convention, the executive committee and Frankel realized they shared a common goal—namely, the establishment of a "larger and more dignified nursing service to the poor and to those of moderate means." What remained unclear was how to achieve this end.[29] To be mutually acceptable, the solution would have to protect the philanthropic activities of VNAs while simultaneously protecting the association's "pay patients" from the stigma of charity. Unfortunately, that perfect solution was never found.[30]

There was something almost magical about that first NOPHN convention. The membership was basking in what one observer described as "the first consciousness of an ego, the buoyancy and hopefulness youth, with growing consciousness of power and unrestricted energy."[31] In her opening address, Wald heralded the NOPHN as an organization where both neophyte and those of experience would work to establish and maintain methods and standards of visiting nursing. This was an organization created not to promote public sentiment or to spread propaganda but in response to cries for help from VNAs across the country. Few organizations, declared Wald, start because of such an obvious need for them.[32]

Fifteen hundred people attended the combined nursing conventions, not only nurses and their board members, but businessmen, doctors, and social workers too.[33] Those present described the atmosphere as permeated by something potent and moving, almost a religious fervor, a "strong emotion and a deep inspiration for service in great forward movement of our generation."[34] Although their meetings had helped crystallize many difficult issues, those who attended returned home confident in their organization's ability to discover the right answers.

By its second annual convention, the NOPHN had progressed from the "husky infant" of Wald's address to a more hazardous developmental stage. The newly elected president, Gardner, told her audience that they should rightfully rejoice in their accomplishments. But history, warned Gardner, "tells us that much self-satisfaction often means death to things of the spirit, a loss of selfless devotion and ultimately an end to progress." Like Jack Horner, the visiting nurses had pulled out many plums, but the movement could not afford to sit in the corner much longer.[35]

By the third convention in 1915, Gardner no longer asked the members of NOPHN to think so metaphorically; nursery rhymes had apparently failed to motivate the membership to deal with what she called "our problem." The focus of Gardner's concern was "a tendency on the part of the nurses to feel that once launched, the [NOPHN] no longer needed the support of their membership." Was it not ironic, queried Gardner, that while laymen and laywomen who had no vote in the organization were assuming an increasing share of its financial burden, nursing's contribution was actually falling off? There were too many important problems awaiting solutions to let this happen. The audience was urged to try to enlarge the membership.[36]

In reality, the NOPEN's total membership was growing, reaching fifteen hundred by the time of the 1915 convention. But unfortunately, the contributions of the members only provided 22 percent of the total annual budget. Financing the organization's work had become the de facto responsibility of the chairmen of the Committee on Membership and Finance. Fortunately, women like Mrs. R. L. Ireland of Cleveland or Mrs. Haughteling of Chicago could be counted on to persuade a sufficient number of "ladies" to support the work of the NOPHN when other fundraising techniques failed.[37]

Like many VNAs, the organization found the demand for its services growing faster than its ability to increase income. The past year had been especially trying financially, for at one point, the NOPHN had actually found itself completely without funds. Ironically, the members of the finance committee were unreachable, since they were all vacationing in New England. In desperation, Crandall was forced to call on one the organization's "staunchest and most wise friends" for advice. Fortunately, she left not only with advice but with enough money to see the organization through until November when some of the "sustaining" memberships were due.[38]

The organization's precarious financial condition had a remarkable effect on the executive committee's ability to examine its needs. First, the committee concluded that every effort would be made to reverse the lack of active support of their fundraising efforts by the New York membership, believing this would help not only raise funds but also add "prestige" to the organization in the east. Second, they concluded that through a systematic effort in every state, they would work to establish "a widely distributed and constantly increasing" active and associate membership. Realizing this would be a slow process, the committee planned to find several more "sustaining" members to supplement their income from regular dues. Finally, the committee would try to find one or more persons willing to provide an endorsement for the NOPHN.[39] Dauntless, the chairman of the finance committee declared this "harassment of too meager support," a temporary embarrassment brought on by "the lack of interest in anything so abstract as this organization's purpose by a public almost hysterical over the war and the invasion of Belgium."[40]

At the suggestion of Wald, it was decided to extend the search for financial support to include the Rockefeller Foundation. Gertrude Peabody, a member of the Boston Instructive District Nursing Association's (IDNA) board, agreed to write to her friend Jerome Green, secretary of the foundation, requesting his personal consideration of the NOPHN's need for support.[41]

In her letter to John D. Rockefeller and her subsequent interview at the foundation, Crandall described the purpose and importance of the NOPHN as well as its need for $2,000 a year for five years. Although the foundation agreed to consider her proposal, it did so with reluctance. The absence of some representative laymen and women on the NOPHN directorate was seen by the foundation as a real problem. It "lent the impression on the public that the organization was chiefly, if not wholly, of and for nurses."[42]

The executive committee quickly recognized their mistake: "Sound principles and good work count," but they had forgotten that "names also have a decided value." Unwilling to jeopardize their affiliation with the American Nurses Association (ANA) by electing lay members to their board, the nurses were obligated to find some less radical solution. After much discussion, the executive committee voted to establish an advisory council of "eminent" men and women: C-E. A. Winslow, William Welch, Herman Biggs, Helen Hartley Jenkins, Julie Lathrop, Mrs. William Vanderbilt, Frankel, and Cyrus McCormick.[43]

The executive committee's gesture proved insufficient. After review of the NOPHN's proposal, Mr. Wickliffe Rose felt unable to recommend an appropriation. His decision was based on the belief that an organization attempting to cover a whole national field on a budget of $9,000 "could not hope to do much more than cultivate public sentiment." He believed the sum requested could and should be raised from individual membership.[44]

No doubt in response to the foundation's decision, Crandall's next annual report assaulted nursing associations' tradition of "closed doors." Lay and professional members should have equal rights, and she urged the membership of the NOPHN to give this question serious thought. It is certainly a contradiction, she pointed out, to ask lay members to contribute four-fifths of the NOPHN's income while accepting only a limited share of control over the organization's policies and programs: "It comes dangerously near to taxation without representation," she declared. But Crandall found insufficient support for her view; lay members continued to give "wise guidance" and money, while the nurse continued to make the decisions.[45]

Despite a rather anemic growth in membership and continuing financial insecurity, by the 1916 convention, the NOPHN could boast of several accomplishments. The newly formed Committee on Education had completed an introductory program in public health nursing for hospital training programs. The committee's intent was not simply to create a course in public health nursing but rather to plan a program of study that made it possible for all nurses to acquire what they called "the social point of view of disease." Despite their concerns with many problems already confronting training schools, the members of the National League for Nursing Education (NLNE) attending the convention unanimously agreed to introduce the committee's recommendation as rapidly as possible into their schools' curricula.[46]

At the same convention, the Committee on Records and Statistics presented their recently completed report. The committee recommended that the nursing record card they had developed be immediately adopted by all VNAs. This, it was emphasized, was simply a first step toward establishing and maintaining uniform standards. The next step, urged Frankel, chairman of the committee, was the adoption of a standardized financial statement. Standardized forms for reporting were essential so that a VNA could begin to make comparisons from year to year and between organizations; in other words, the time had come to begin to evaluate their successes and failures.[47]

Finally, Crandall could claim that as a result of her visits covering 32,021 miles to sixty-three cities, to eighty-three public addresses, and to ninety-one conferences, a vital spark had been applied to the "latent force within many and varied communities." In a number of cities, public health nursing had been reorganized and extended; health work had been separated from charities; the standards of work, workers, and records had been improved; new associations had been organized; and a division of public health nursing had been established in a state department of health as the result of Crandall's efforts that year.[48]

II

The founding of the NOPHN had not been the only significant visiting nurse event of the June 1912 nursing convention; it was simply the most conspicuous. Sharing the limelight was Jane Delano's announcement that the Red Cross was planning to form a Rural Nursing Service and would be seeking visiting nurses to enter this new field.[49] Unmistakably, the nursing leadership had not restricted their efforts to protect and promote the future of visiting nursing to the activities of the NOPHN.[50]

While working to establish the NOPHN with its primarily urban focus, several of the same women were simultaneously creating a separate organization to promote visiting nursing in rural communities. Even though the Rural Nursing Service was affiliated with the Red Cross, everyone, according to Beard, was "interested in having them closely connected with visiting nurse associations instead of following the tendency to be Red Cross and only that and exclusively that."[51]

A concern for improving country life was not peculiar to the visiting nurse, and not surprisingly, the cast of characters sharing their desire to uplift rural life was remarkably similar to that already encountered by the visiting nurse in the city.[52] While, in 1908, President Roosevelt was contributing to what one author dubbed the "general bucolic excitement" by appointing his Country Life Commission, Wald was busily promoting visiting nursing's contribution to this scheme—the "country nurse."[53]

Wald's goal was to create "an extensive and systematically organized service to nursing [for] the sick country person" under the auspices of the American Red Cross. Rural nursing would, she argued, provide the Red Cross a peacetime mission, saving the society from the disorganization and loss of enthusiasm unavoidable during periods of inactivity between emergencies. Jacob Schiff, a member of the Board of Incorporation of the American Red Cross and who had already made substantial contributions to work at Henry Street Settlement, supported her scheme.[54]

Unfortunately, when Schiff presented Wald's proposal for country nursing at the December 1910 meeting of the board, most members failed to share his enthusiasm. The only outcome was the appointment of a subcommittee to talk the matter over with Wald. But majority opinion was quickly swayed at the next annual meeting when Schiff and Mrs. Whitelaw Reid offered to provide the money necessary to begin such a rural health nursing service.[55]

A special committee was immediately appointed, which quickly recommended approval of the project for rural nursing, suggesting a trial year be conducted under the supervision of the Committee on Rural Nursing. The committee's members were already well-known to Wald and her nursing colleagues. Mabel Boardman, who chaired the committee, Mrs. William Draper, and Reid were all prominent members of the Washington, DC, and New York societies. Although they worked as volunteers, they had a great deal of influence over their societies and were strong supporters of nurses of a "professional caliber." Other members of the committee included John Glenn of the Russell Sage Foundation; Rose of the Rockefeller Foundation; Winfred Smith, superintendent of the Johns Hopkins Hospital; and Dr. J. W. Schereschewsky of the Public Health Service. The nurses on the committee were Wald, Goodrich, and Delano.[56]

At the first meeting held in November 1912, the nurse members of the committee were given the task of making recommendations for the nursing service. Taking advantage of this opportunity, they immediately convinced the committee that due to the nature of the rural nurse's work, she must possess the highest qualifications. Their suggestions included requiring not only all applicants to complete a four-month course of training under the supervision of a recognized VNA but also the development of scholarships and loan funds necessary to make this a plausible requirement. The committee's rapid acceptance of the nurses' recommendations suggested that, at least for the moment, the Rural Nursing Service would be allowed to develop under the careful control and protection of the nursing leadership.[57]

The appointment of Fannie Clements as superintendent for the nursing service heightened their enthusiasm. Clements was young, but by training and experience, she was amply fitted to organize this new work. A native of Massachusetts, she was a graduate of Smith College, Boston City Hospital School for Nursing, and Boston Lying-In Hospital. She had experience in private-duty and district nursing and had worked in the social service department of the Boston Dispensary while completing her studies at the School for Social Workers. She epitomized the visiting nurse's nurse.[58]

The original plan for the Rural Nursing Service was not to employ nurses but to "promote and popularize" the idea of affiliation between the Red Cross and local boards of health or associations. Affiliation meant the Red Cross would provide a "properly qualified nurse" and give her guidance and supervision, while the local group would provide her salary.[59]

Clements quickly discovered that her most fundamental problem would be finding qualified nurses. Not only were there few public health nurses at the time, but even fewer met the Red Cross standards; fewer still had any experience in rural nursing. At the time, only six VNAs offered postgraduate training and none taught rural nursing.[60] By October 1913, Teachers College, in cooperation with the Henry Street Settlement and the Westchester District Nursing Association, had initiated a four-month course specifically planned to meet the needs of the Red Cross.[61]

By the end of 1913, sixteen nurses had been appointed. They were employed by visiting nurse committees, nursing associations, Red Cross chapters, public health leagues, civic clubs, and antituberculosis societies. Growth was rapid enough to require the appointment of a supervisor to assist Clements, and the name was changed to Town and Country Nursing Service so that services could be extended to "small communities, not strictly rural."[62]

The same year, in an effort to formalize a cooperative relationship between the four nursing organizations, Crandall, representing the NOPHN, Adelaide Nutting, representing the National League Nursing Education, and Mathild Kruger, representing the ANA, were added to the Town and Country Nursing Service Committee. Dock would later describe this as a great achievement, making "American nurses a real power."[63]

By May of 1913, Wald successfully negotiated a cooperative agreement between the Red Cross and the MLI. The Red Cross agreed to provide nursing care for the company's industrial policyholders, while the Metropolitan agreed to endorse the regulations authorized for rural nurses by the Red Cross. As a result, the company was able to effortlessly extend nursing services to many more of its policyholders. Over time, many local associations survived solely on the basis of the Metropolitan payments, which represented a reliable and often increasing source of income.[64]

By December of 1913, concerns about the "the delicate questions of coordination" had arisen, which, according to Wald, required immediate attention. As a preventive measure, Wald suggested a meeting between NOPHN and the Town and Country Nursing Service. Her goal was to produce an agreement as to each organization's "distinctive place" and a plan for how it could "interlock without overlapping."[65]

Anticipating the expansionist tendencies of Boardman and other members of the Town and Country Nursing Service Committees, Wald hoped to curtail any growth that would result in competition with the NOPHN. With that concern in mind, she wrote Reid, the chair of the Town and Country Nursing Committee, expressing her belief that "it would be practical and statesmanlike for . . . the Red Cross to limit its work during its constructive period to the . . . promotion of interest in country nursing, and the establishment and supervision of nurses in country communities and small towns." She also suggested the Red Cross not establish educational centers but continue to send nurses to the established centers provided by other organizations, leaving to Teachers College and the NOPHN the business of promoting education for public health nurses. The NOPHN was, according to Wald, a society "for education and mutual benefit, a union of workers and those interested in their work," while the work of the Red Cross was "administrative and supervisory."[66] Since the same people were interested in both organizations, it seemed reasonable to assume that they could meet and, with little difficulty, define the relationship between the two organizations. Wald's meeting took place in Washington, DC, in March 1914 and produced what would be the first of several such nonaggression pacts.[67]

Despite the hopes of many, the Town and Country Nursing Service remained a modest undertaking. By 1917, eighty-nine affiliations with a total of ninety-seven nurses had been established in twenty-one states. The earliest programs were initiated in eastern states and then the South and Midwest. Prior to World War I, there were only five affiliations west of the Mississippi. In the aggregate, the work of the Red Cross nurse mirrored that of the visiting nurse in most urban settings. The majority of cases (47 percent) required bedside care of the sick, while 8 percent were visits to schoolchildren, 10 percent infant welfare, 2 percent prenatal, 3 percent tuberculosis, 4 percent sanitary inspection, and the remainder "business and unclassified" calls. While the rural nurse cared for fewer patients than the visiting nurse in the city, they tended to make more visits to each patient.[68]

III

The renewed harmony between NOPHN and the Red Cross was short-lived. Ironically, it was Wald's pacifist stance that placed the first wedge in their relationship. The initial conflict was over Wald's efforts to convince the executive committee of the NOPHN to publicly denounce the war and the sending of American Red Cross nurses to aid Europe in September 1914.[69] Delano vigorously opposed this proposal, reminding the executive committee that the Red Cross was under treaty obligations to send relief to other countries when needed, adding that she considered it rather presumptive "for a small body of nurses to publicly criticize an international organization such as the Red Cross, which had received the world's highest endorsement since 1864."[70]

While agreeing with the wisdom of Delano's suggestions, the executive committee and, according to Crandall, "others of their standing" no longer shared her sentiments for the Red Cross.[71] As far as they were concerned, the Red Cross and especially the Town and Country Nursing Service were in need of assistance. They strongly felt, declared Crandall, "that the work [was] not credible, let alone magnificent" and could no longer feel justified in recommending affiliation with the Red Cross to small communities in the vicinity of their own cities: "Owing to the natural tendency of the small communities to call on" the larger VNAs in the vicinity for their "guidance and help," the Red Cross, as a Washington-based organization, created an artificial arrangement simply pretending to provide these communities with supervision and guidance.[72]

Delano's assessment of the situation was, not surprisingly, just the opposite. As soon as the United States entered the war, she and Clements met with Crandall to request a "tentative curtailment of the work of the national organization in favor of the Red Cross Town and Country Nursing Service." Specifically, the NOPHN should no longer reply to letters from communities with populations of less than twenty-five thousand, forwarding such letters instead to the Red Cross. At the same meeting, Delano raised certain objections, in light of the demands of war, to the standards for nursing service suggested by the NOPHN.[73] While they were willing to admit that the services of the two organizations often overlapped, the NOPHN concluded that the suggested limitations could not be justified even temporarily. Certainly, the demands of war had not so accelerated the needs for nurses to justify lowering their hard-won standards.[74]

Their refusal to comply with Delano's suggestions was presented at the April 28, 1917, meeting of the Red Cross National Committee on Nursing Service. In a brief statement, they acknowledged the administrative services rendered by the Red Cross in small towns and rural communities but concluded that the NOPHN could not "in the nature of its purposes and obligations, limited its operations either geographically or professionally."[75]

A second area of conflict between the two organizations was how best to meet the military's need for nurses. The American Red Cross, eager to fulfill its obligation as the procurement agency for the army and the navy, initiated a massive recruitment effort aimed at all nurses regardless of field of employment. The Red Cross plan sent the NOPHN into a panic, for if successful, the country would be depleted of its finest public health nurses.[76]

The NOPHN's analysis of the country's wartime needs for nurses produced a different and conflicting set of priorities: "Young graduates strong and fresh from a modern surgical training" should be sent, argued Beard, "to man the wards of the field hospitals," while the public health nurse should stay home. According to the NOPHN's analysis, the Red Cross should issue a "pronouncement" recognizing the public health nurse's efforts to conserve the nation's health as a patriotic service equal to military duty, calling them for service aboard only as a last resort.[77] Not surprisingly, Delano rejected the NOPHN suggestions, which they had chosen to "very carefully" discuss at the April 28 meeting.[78]

Public health nurses had no intention of allowing Delano or her international organization to stand in their way. The opportunities presented by the war were too great to tolerate such interference. As Beard reminded her audience at the 1917 nursing convention, "the future was big with promise."[79] Not surprisingly, the war greatly increased the confidence and self-image not only of public health nurses but of the American nurse in general. It gave them opportunities and contacts never before accessible, and they intended to demonstrate what they could do once given the chance.[80]

The public health nursing leadership was confident that the public would demand their services as never before, that health officers would beg them to remain at their posts and later, after the war, public health nurses "qualified by education and experience" would be called for everywhere as never before. Under such circumstances, allowing the Red Cross to call for duly qualified and more experienced public health nurses would inevitably result in their replacement by inferior substitutes. The results would be disastrous. Thus the NOPHN chose for its focus for 1917 a nationwide program to recruit nurses for public health work and a campaign to obtain nationwide recognition of their contribution to the war.[81]

Crandall wrote the VNAs across the country, requesting they "persuade every public health nurse that the largest patriotic service she could render was to remain at her post."[82] Having failed in their efforts to obtain a "pronouncement" from the Red Cross, the advisory council decided to direct its campaign at a higher authority, the Council of National Defense. They chose a three-part strategy. First, Winslow wrote Drs. Welch, Biggs, Rupert Blue, and Simon Flexner, proposing, in the name of the advisory council of the NOPHN, that a nurse be added to the Council of National Defense. Second, letters of introduction from Welch and Biggs were obtained for Beard and Crandall to Franklin Martin, chairman of the General Medical Board of the Council of National Defense. Finally, Biggs and Welch took their proposition to the general medical board and "urged that very serious and prompt attention be given it because of its great importance."[83]

The proposal was then referred to Surgeon General Blue's committee for further study, and a conference between representatives of the NOPHN and the Red Cross was authorized. As a result, a subcommittee on public health nursing of the Committee on Hygiene and Sanitation of the General Medical Board of the Council of National Defense was formed. Not surprisingly, Beard was appointed chair of the subcommittee.[84] Of the members initially appointed by Blue, Beard was the only public health nurse, but at her request, Crandall and Gardner were added to the committee. The committee's charge was to analyze the effects of war on community health in Europe, examine the status of community health at home, monitor changing conditions produced by war, and if necessary, create plans for the extension of community health work.[85]

Not surprisingly, at the June 18, 1917, meeting of the subcommittee on public health nursing, Delano, herself a member, read a letter she was sending to local communities advising them to exercise special care in calling from their regular duties administrators and teachers in hospitals and schools of nursing and public health nurses. In three months, the NOPHN had obtained its "pronouncement." In reality, though, Delano's letter came as a great relief, since it had become clear that they would not be able to obtain unanimous support for their "pronouncement" from the General Medical Board.[86]

That same month, a meeting of leading nurses resulted in the creation of the National Emergency Committee on Nursing, with Nutting as chair. The purpose of the committee was to ensure an adequate supply of nurses at home and a future supply for both home and military use. Opposed to any method of increasing the supply of nurses that threatened the standards of nursing or nursing education, the instigators of the committee—Wald, Nutting, Crandall, and Stewart—carefully selected additional members who shared their concerns. By the end of June, through the efforts of Welch, the services of the committee were accepted by the General Medical Board. Nutting's committee, as it was known, became the National Committee on Nursing of the General Medical Board. Remarkably, the General Medical Board generally backed the stands taken by Nutting's committee, even when, on occasion, this action caused friction with the war department or the Red Cross.[87]

The nursing members of Nutting's committee also served on the Committee on Red Cross Nursing and Wald's Committee on Home Nursing. Wald's committee came under the section on sanitation of the Committee of Labor of the Council of National Defense and was created to promote public health nursing services for industrial workers throughout the country.[88] The three nursing committees accepted the NOPHN's offer to send Crandall to Washington, DC, to serve as their secretary on a full-time basis.[89] After arriving in Washington, Crandall was made a member of the office staff of the Medical Section of the Council of National Defense, which provided her with an office, office equipment, and secretarial help.[90] In addition to paying Crandall's salary and expenses, the NOPHN also contributed $5,750 to help finance the initial work of the three nursing committees. Mary Lent, the assistant executive secretary of the NOPHN, took over the NOPHN's other activities in the New York office.[91]

By the end of July 1917 Beard, resident of the NOPHN, could declare that everything the public health nurses had tried to secure and "even a great deal more" had come to pass. Their "pronouncement" had been obtained from the Red Cross, the work of their committees was "dove-tailing splendidly," all their programs had been initiated, and "much respect" was being shown to them by the officers. Clearly, she concluded, "a great opportunity to serve undoubtedly lies before us."[92]

The NOPHN felt further exalted when Lent was selected as the supervising nurse for what were called the extracontainment zones. These were the zones surrounding the fifty-one military camps established in the United States during World War I and varying in size from five miles to one hundred miles. Their purpose was to protect soldiers and their families from the health hazards of the surrounding community: disease, poor housing, inadequate sewage disposal, contaminated milk and water, and venereal disease. The cost of this "sanitary effort" was shared by the Red Cross ($507,000), state and local health departments ($650,000), and the U.S. Public Health Service ($1,201,900).[93]

Lent's ability to create a nationwide standardized nursing service was highly valued by the NOPHN. Not only did it give the public health nurse high visibility in new regions of the country, but it also placed her services where the NOPHN believed they belonged—as an integral part of a government-supported "unified health service." No doubt the NOPHN's support of the development of public health nursing within the Public Health Service and state departments of health was in part an expression of their fears of the expansionist tendencies of the Red Cross.

Recognizing that a large proportion of their success was the result of putting a full-time representative in Washington, DC, the NOPHN began to seek additional income to support their expensive "war services." Early in October 1917, Beard, through the assistance of one of the Boston association's board members, arranged a meeting with George Vincent of the Rockefeller Foundation.[94] The NOPHN's second request for financial assistance encountered a much more receptive review from the foundation. Beard was described by the foundation staff in glowing terms, while the NOPHN was characterized as "a well directed and well manned organization" that had something valuable and something already valued to offer the field of public health. Apparently, the NOPHN's activities related to the Council of National Defense had not gone without notice by the foundation and measurably influenced their favorable decision.[95] The foundation agreed to provide $15,000 to NOPHN in 1918, $10,000 in 1919, and $5,000 in 1920. Their intent was not to make permanent contributions to the NOPHN "but rather to give aid during an experimental period in which it is hoped that the work can be put upon a basis where its revenues from various committees together with the subscription of its clientele will give adequate support."[96]

Beard described the war as both a crisis and a challenge for public health nursing, for it was accompanied by both opportunities and responsibilities.[97] In fact, the war did have a significant impact on most health departments and VNAs. As doctors and nurses joined the military, the visiting nurse found herself supplementing the work of the remaining doctors and taking the place of the private-duty nurse in many homes.[98]

The wartime experiences of the IDNA of Boston illustrated the impact felt by many of the larger urban associations as a result of the war. In 1917, the Boston association employed seventy nurses; by 1918, the demand for nurses was so great that not only had the staff grown to one hundred, but it was also necessary for each nurse to make fewer visits to each patient while caring for a larger number of patients. This growth in volume of work, not surprisingly, produced a comparable growth in the annual budget from $90,634 in 1917 to $125,779 in 1918.[99] At the end of the year, the board of directors declared that never in its history had their organization faced such "monstrous and difficult" problems. Like the Providence association, whose director (Gardner) was in Italy, Boston had done so without the guidance of Beard, who was "on loan" for NOPHN work in Washington, DC.[100]

At the Red Cross's call for nurses for foreign service, many of the most experienced visiting nurses in the country volunteered, and many more would have gone had they not been ineligible because of foreign birth or failure to pass the physical exam.[101] Since a large percent of most VNA staffs were enrolled in the Red Cross, the staff shortage would have become even more severe had it not been for the Red Cross "pronouncement" requesting public health nurses to stay in this country.[102]

Staff were also resigning for less than "patriotic reasons." According to the Philadelphia lady managers, the nurses were beginning to realize that as a result of the war, "many places were now open to them, and this [did] not lend to their stability on any staff." The managers concluded that the best they could hope for was to make the nurses feel a "greater responsibility" to the association.[103] VNAs used a variety of methods to deal with the decreasing supply of nurses and the increasing demand for care. In Philadelphia, not only did the managers try to increase the staff's sense of responsibility; they did the same with their patients' families. Patients were taught to seek care only when absolutely necessary, while their families were taught to provide more of the care.[104]

Some associations began to try to convince larger numbers of training schools to send more senior pupils for longer periods of time both for "selfish reasons and as a public service." Thus the VNAs would provide the student nurses training, room, and board, and in exchange, the students would have the benefit of their services without having to pay them a salary.[105] Many associations were forced for the first time to hire married nurses, and some began to give serious thought to using both trained and untrained attendants and volunteers under the supervision of their nursing staff.[106]

The Philadelphia association, for example, was eager to use volunteers in homes for health teaching but first sought the advice of the NOPHN, hoping it might "be possible to develop some nationwide policy" that would maintain standards while simultaneously meeting the increasing staff needs of the associations.[107] Two days later, the executive committee of the NOPHN met but decided they would take "no action or stand" on the subject of volunteer workers.[108] Unlike Nutting's Committee on Nursing, which emphatically disapproved of the use of nonprofessional workers, they believed that if given proper training and supervision, they would prove useful. But the executive committee, unwilling to make such an opinion public, instead encouraged the use of attendants and volunteers by the Philadelphia, Boston, and Providence associations on an experimental basis. Thus in essence, the national organization advised the local associations to proceed by whatever method they thought best.[109]

Simultaneously, health departments, unable to cope with the accelerated demand for health workers, were inventing their own experimental programs with nonnurse workers. One such plan, which was supported by Haven Emerson, Commissioner of Health for New York City, involved the use of a new type of nonnurse worker who would be trained to do the preventive and educational portion of public health visiting. In this plan, only the bedside care of the sick would remain under the aegis of public health nurses.[110]

Emerson discussed his proposal with Nutting in July of 1917, and by the end of the month, Nutting, in turn, had shared the proposal with nurses across the country. Although sympathetic with the emergency situation that had precipitated Emerson's action, the nurses who responded found his solution unacceptable. On August 1, 1917, Emerson wrote Nutting expressing appreciation for her painstaking inquiry and her suggestions for an alternative course. The above notwithstanding, Emerson told Nutting that he had decided to go ahead "to try, in a modest way, . . . a course for the preparation of public health workers, based upon higher educational requirements than those usually demanded by the nurses' training schools, the course to take two years and be planned along radically different lines from those at present followed, or likely to be followed, while nurses are prepared under the auspices of training schools."

Graduates would work under the supervision of nurses or doctors, and since, according to Emerson, they probably would not remain very long in service, their salary would consequently be small—$700–$750 per year. Thus Emerson hoped to provide in half the time and at a significant savings a worker who would be prepared to meet the health department's exact specifications.[111]

Because he was removed from office when a Tammany administration was elected in January 1918, Emerson was unable to implement his plan. But he was not alone in his interest in developing nonnurse public health workers. Courses for college graduates similar to the one Emerson had proposed were being suggested in Wisconsin, California, and Virginia; in France, the Rockefeller Foundation's Committee for Tuberculosis and the American Red Cross Children's Bureau were establishing a ten-month course for health visitors.[112]

The assault came from both far and near, but probably the most distressing was the announcement by Biggs, a member of the NOPHN's own advisory council, that he too believed that "unprofessional women should be trained as health visitors for public health work rather than nurses."[113] At roughly the same time, Dr. John Dill Robertson, commissioner of health in Chicago, formulated what he thought was an even better idea. Believing, as did many physicians, that any bright, competent woman could be trained for nursing in a few months, Robertson decided to take advantage of what he called the "auspicious times" to establish a new school. It was called the Chicago Training School for Home and Public Health Nursing and claimed to be able to produce a capable nurse in two months, on 4,231 of them in the first year. Trained nurses feared Robertson's panacea would hurt the profession and later found great delight in telling the story of a woman who called up one of the Chicago hospitals and said she had illness in her family and wanted a good nurse, adding, "Don't send me on of them public health nurses, as I am one myself."[114]

But Robertson's proposal, combined with Emerson's plan and other developments actually underway, led many public health nurses to become alarmed in 1918. A nurse from Virginia expressed their concern with unusual clarity when she said, "In other words, the college women were to take over the highest functions of the nurse, those of teacher and leader, after a brief 'course' as though these highest functions were so little technical that they might be laid in a few months as a durable veneer upon the foundation of a college education. This idea expanded would strip from the nursing profession the field of public health and lower the dignity of the bedside care of the sick."

Even Vincent of the Rockefeller Foundation, who approached the problem from a different perspective, believed that unless the nursing profession found a suitable way to prepare public health nurses in large numbers, they were certain to be replaced by nonnurse health visitors.[115]

Opposed to the idea of a health visitor without formal nurse training, organized public health nurses were at last forced to publicly support the use of aids or attendants. If a partially trained woman was needed, it was argued, her place should be at the bedside of convalescent and chronic patients, where she could be supervised by a highly trained nurse. The creation of an assistant whose activities nursing could control through licensure, training, and supervision was far less threatening than the continued growth of a new competitive profession.[116]

At the 1918 nursing convention, the time had finally come to stop considering alternatives and to take action. Gardner reminded her audience that the attendant who for many years was "non-existent in the eyes of most of us" had more recently become for the public health nurse more like the line of battledore in the game of battledore and shuttlecock. At the business meeting of the NOPHN membership, the board of directors submitted a resolution proposing a "code" for the use of workers with less than standard training in associations with severe shortages of nurses. The resolution passed and the code was published in the July 1918 issue of the *Public Health Nurse Quarterly* (*PHNQ*).[117] The NOPHN planned to work with the NLNE to develop an educational course for attendants, vowing to "stand man to man with the League in upholding standards"[118]

The board of directors also agreed that as an emergency measure, they would allow "a grave concession to its standards for preparation" and approve an emergency training course of ten weeks for nurses; but only those "guaranteed the close supervision of a well-qualified public health nurse after they are placed at work in the community."[119] Ironically, at the same convention, Goodrich convinced the nurses attending the joint session of the three nursing organizations to protect the professional status of nursing by opposing the Red Cross plan to use volunteer nurse aids in military hospitals.[120]

In the meantime, Bolton, who had joined her husband in Washington, DC, decided to take on nursing as her contribution to the war.[121] This was, she reminded the executive committee of the NOPHN, "the chance of the age to start a far reaching and thoroughly aggressive campaign." Determined that money would not impede the NOPHN's progress, she formed her own financial aid committee, the Emergency War Finance Committee. She urged the executive committee to "increase the budget to meet new opportunities," and her committee would assume all responsibility for any expenses beyond that covered by the Rockefeller Foundation grant.[122] The NOPHN was "for the first time in its history, freed . . . from the bondage of poverty," declared Crandall.[123] In response to their newfound wealth, the library services for the members were expanded, an educational secretary was hired to advise agencies and postgraduate programs, and a Chicago office was opened. During the year, plans were initiated to open two more offices: one in Portland and the other in Atlanta.[124]

Within a few months of initiating her war efforts on behalf of nursing, Bolton had produced a study of what she called "the machinery" of the NOPHN. She concluded that to increase the organization's efficiency, it was necessary to do away with the "present artificial character" of the executive committee, which was the result of having lay members who could not vote but "whose contributions not only to the meetings but to the association [were] of a specialized character and therefore especially valuable." She insisted that a more proper division of responsibilities be initiated: laypeople who are contributing their money, their interest, and their time should have a voice in the executive sessions of the organization. That voice, she declared, "should never be so large as to dominate, but it should be heard." She assured the executive committee that lay members would "take the utmost care not to overstep our bounds." She realized that although this ridiculous situation existed because of the NOPHN's desire to conform to the wishes of the ANA, it could no longer continue. Public health nurses must remember that unlike general nursing, their field was, from its inception, the direct result of the united action of lay and professional people. Bolton and her committee of Cleveland ladies believed that the time had come to amend the bylaws of the NOPHN.[125]

There was a good deal of validity in Bolton's criticism. Obviously, when only 10 percent of the NOPHN budget came from memberships, laymen and laywomen were largely responsible for its existence. Once this issue had been so clearly articulated, the nurses were forced to choose between conforming to the ANA's "closed door" policy toward lay board members or risk antagonizing their lay contributors. Bolton's proposal was first discussed in September 1918 by the executive committee of the NOPHN. Agreement was unanimous that Bolton, with the assistance of the staff, should redraft the bylaws for presentation to the entire board. At a special session early in October, the board of directors unanimously approved the proposed amendments. As there would be no general meeting of the membership until 1920, they voted to call an emergency session of the NOPHN for December 13 and 14 in Chicago.[126]

In her editorial the next month, Beard expressed her disappointment that it had not been possible to give the members more opportunity to consider the proposed changes but that those few (sixty) members able to attend this special session made the change in bylaws "necessary to the efficient management of the organization." Beard went on to tell her readers that Friday 13, 1918, "will go down in the history of public health nursing as a Red Letter date, for it was unanimously voted at the general session . . . to elect four nonprofessional members to the Directorate of the NOPHN. Ever since that other historic Chicago meeting of 1912 when the national organization was formed, public health nurses have felt the need of this." The new members of the board included Bolton and Mrs. Lowman from Cleveland, Mrs. Cudahy from Chicago, and Miss Railey from New Orleans.[127]

The midwestern focus was apparently intentional, for Beard's editorial went on to mention the NOPHN's new Chicago office, their new western board members, and the continued residence of "their official organ," the *PHN* in Cleveland. Surely, suggested Beard, "we shall have a much more general and active development of interest in the national organization, a development which will be more representative geographically as well as in point of numbers, for some of our most important work will have its center in a location more available for western members."[128]

In the interim, the war had virtually halted the growth of the Town and Country Nursing Service. In April 1918, Clements resigned and was eventually replaced by Elizabeth Fox. While the war checked the growth of public health nursing, it simultaneously created conditions that made expansion an inevitable outcome of its conclusion.[129] According to Fox, the war taught people how to organize and accomplish things. They became public-spirited and found "that there are many things more interesting outside their homes than inside." Across the country, communities had organized Red Cross chapters—240 of them—and Fox had every reason to believe that when their war duties were completed, these chapters could be encouraged to turn their attention to "some form of community service"—namely, public health nursing.[130] Having just taken on her new job, Fox, "full of zest," wrote a friend that "we have good reason to think the service is going to develop very rapidly, . . . everything is going to tend our way when the war is over and even is coming that way now."[131]

Anticipating the future, the National Committee of the Red Cross voted in May of 1918 to change their title from Town and Country Nursing Service to Bureau of Public Health Nursing and to remove any restrictions on the size of communities in which Red Cross public health nurses might be employed.[132] The NOPHN viewed these developments with dismay. Crandall contended that the Red Cross leadership, especially Noyes, was developing plans for the future of public health nursing with "exasperating independence and indifference to the special interest and previous experience" of the NOPHN. Crandall even found herself constantly "obliged to keep up the equally irritating process of checking up on the Red Cross in matters of so great importance as the printing of letterheads, applications and credential forms."[133]

Although Crandall "emphatically resented" these activities on the part of the Red Cross, she felt compelled to "endure and submit in silence," at least for the duration of the war. While limiting herself to merely acting as a "thorn in the flesh of them" whenever possible, she vowed the NOPHN would continue to guard the field of public health nursing from the menace of the power of the Red Cross.[134]

Some means needed to be found to limit the ambitions of the Red Cross to "simple experimentation and demonstrations in public health nursing." Apparently, to the NOPHN leadership, the U.S. Public Health Service and state departments of public health provided a promising alternative to the Red Cross. Not surprisingly then, Crandall would, at the close of the war, describe Lent's work with these organizations as "unquestionably the greatest single war service rendered by the NOPHN to the government and to the public—its permanent influence is incalculable."[135]

While privately and anxiously attempting to guard the field of public health nursing from the ruthlessness of their Red Cross competitors, the NOPHN was publicly basking in the glory of its success. At the "wartime convention," as the meeting in the summer of 1918 was dubbed, public health nurses from across the country had the opportunity to recount their year of success as one filled with "great venture, great achievement and great plans."[136]

When the war ended, public health nursing looked to the future with great anticipation, confident that they had earned their place in the new health-care system that would surely evolve. The war had had a tremendous impact on the medical profession, serving as an intensive refresher course for many outdated general practitioners.[137] The practice of medicine would never be the same, and the NOPHN was already preparing for the opportunities for nurses that would follow.

Public health nursing was confident that its efforts to protect the civilian population during the war, its cooperation with the Children's Year Program of the Federal Children's Bureau, and its "self-sacrificing" service during the epidemic of 1918 helped create an unprecedented standing with the public. Furthermore, the shocking findings of the draft had opened many eyes to the need for preventive and health education work with the country's youth, and visiting nursing was, of course, indispensable to such work.[138] Operating under such an assumption meant that the major task facing the NOPHN was to supply the needs of every city requesting the services of a public health nurse. Fortuitously, since ten thousand nurses would be coming back from overseas to find that "the communities have gotten along without them," the solution seemed simple. With "just a little training," these nurses could be encouraged to enter a "new field of usefulness"—public health nursing.[139] Finally, the Rockefeller Foundation had agreed to conduct a study of public health nursing, which the nursing leadership hoped would do for nursing what the Flexner Report had done for medicine.[140]

The 1918 annual report of the Philadelphia association aptly described this period as a "terrific test from which had come both tremendous exhilaration as well as many lessons." The report concluded that "like steel passing through the final test by fire, the society has come forth infinitely stronger than ever before with a new vigor and redoubled strength. The staff, the board of managers and the public have discovered new possibilities, both in themselves and in each other and are entering upon the years to come with a united purpose gained through the terrible and wonderful experiences shared together."[141]

The NOPHN, no doubt, shared the sentiments of the Philadelphia society. The conflicts since 1912 had forged strong bonds and shared visions between NOPHN and visiting nurses, their lady managers, and even the MLI. Interestingly, what had been lost was their allegiance to the dogma and ways of the nursing profession in general and the Red Cross in particular. Public health nurses had entered what Mary Roberts later described as "that long period during which considerably more emphasis was placed on public health than upon nursing."[142]

Chapter 5

The Decline of Public Health Nursing

Economical and Pragmatic but
No Longer Necessary

For visiting nurse associations (VNAs), the Red Cross, and the National Organization for Public Health Nursing (NOPHN), the decade of the 1920s began
with great hopes. The future could not have seemed more promising. Even
before the nursing leadership could return home from their wartime activities,
the Rockefeller Foundation had legitimated their value by initiating a major
study of the field that would, it seemed likely, prove a catalyst for considerable
positive reform. At home, the nurses found community support for their work
equally gratifying. Although briefly delayed by a postwar shortage of nurses,
the number and size of public health nursing organizations rapidly expanded
across the country.

Ironically, having created these new programs, many voluntary organizations found themselves unable to raise the money to support them. Deficits
and contracting budgets more often than not followed. While self-analysis
produced volumes of reports and ambitious conclusions, what followed were
modest solutions, halfheartedly implemented. Examined from any perspective,
the circumstances that had created the need for these nurses earlier in the century now simply no longer existed.

Publicly funded public health nursing programs offered the only ray of
hope in this otherwise dismal set of circumstances. While all other public
health nursing programs retrenched and remodeled, these flourished until they
eventually dominated the whole field. But these organizations created a very
different kind of reality for the public health nurse. Unlike the VNAs or the Red
Cross programs, where nurses and ladies had created a domain of their own,
these organizations belonged to health officers or superintendents of education.

The policies, programs, and organizations that resulted shared little in common with those of voluntary public health nursing agencies. By the end of the decade, there was little similarity in what nurses actually did across this disparate group of organizations, although all still laid claim to the title of public health nurse.

All did share common problems. With the end of immigration, the growing importance of the hospital, and the declining significance of infectious diseases, all public health nurses found their work relegated to an increasingly marginal role in the health-care system. How and why a movement that might have been significant in delivering comprehensive health care to the public failed will be the focus of this chapter.

I

In December of 1918, the Rockefeller Foundation called a meeting to address some of the questions raised by the wartime need for public health nurses. The nursing leadership was delighted, realizing that if wartime plans to use less expensive nonnurse workers were continued in peacetime, the once multifaceted role of the public health nurse would be severely constricted. The foundation hoped that a conference might serve as a first step toward the kind of consensus that would result in an improved and unifying paradigm for public health nursing. As anticipated, the meeting dealt with a variety of questions, but no consensus could be reached. Consequently, a committee was nominated by ballot to study the questions raised at the meeting. Those elected included William Welch, Herman Biggs, C.-E. A. Winslow, Mary Beard, Annie Goodrich, Adelaide Nutting, and Lillian Wald.[1]

Even before the new committee could meet, expressions of concern about its potential effectiveness were received by the foundation. Critics who characterized the "nursing trust" as narrow, shortsighted, and selfish were appalled to find the nurses' views represented 4 to 3 on the committee. The whole question of public health nursing required a more progressive point of view, they claimed, than these "rather old stagers in nursing" were capable of producing.[2]

In contrast, the nurses could not have been more pleased with this outcome: "A great hope is growing in my heart," wrote Nutting to Winslow, chair of the committee, "for the future of our cherished work—what a wonderful thing it would be if the Winslow Committee could do for nursing what the Flexner Report" did for medicine.[3]

No doubt in an effort to appear impartial on this surprisingly controversial subject, four nonnurses were added to the committee at its first meeting: Livingston Farrand, William Holt, Mrs. Isabel Lowman, and Julia Lathrop. Even

though the balance of power on the committee gave the appearance of having radically shifted, all were, in fact, supporters of the views of the "nursing
trust." By that summer, the foundation had provided $20,000 to fund a study of
public health nursing, and Josephine Goldmark reluctantly agreed to conduct
it. Confident that this important investigation had been placed in competent
and friendly hands, the nursing leadership could at last turn to other long-
interrupted matters.[4]

At home, the VNAs were just beginning to return to normal. At last
relieved of the strain of constantly facing new difficulties with a staff and
administration depleted by calls for war service or by the flu epidemics of
1918 and 1919, most associations planned to take up their normal activities
with renewed vigor and unprecedented community support. Unfortunately,
1919 proved an unexpectedly difficult year. The accumulated weariness of
the staff and the continued shortage of qualified public health nurses delayed
most plans for yet another year.[5]

The nursing shortage was not simply a residual effect of the war but also
a reflection of the competitive efforts of health departments, local Red Cross
chapters, and VNAs to attract enough staff to expand old programs and initiate new ones.[6] According to one analysis of the shortage, nursing's attitude of
endurance and self-deprivation had been at once its hallmark and its stigma,
but the laws of supply and demand had begun to alter such attitudes. Obviously, self-preservation and opportunity both dictated that nurses seek those
positions offering the greatest rewards. Accordingly, many VNAs were forced
to examine what, beyond prestige, they had to offer.[7]

When at last fully aware of the choices confronting them, the boards of
the larger VNAs reluctantly began to give the financial position of the public
health nurse serious consideration. Boards traditionally resisted any attempt
salaries, explained Mrs. Lowman, because they viewed them holding in trust
"public funds" and were thus obligated to protect their treasury from unnecessary spending. All would unconsciously attempt to delay a decision in the matter, she continued, by finding out what other cities of similar size were paying
their nurses. After all, operating "somewhat upon the principle that what is
must be right," they had been able over the years to guarantee a certain degree
of order and security that would be unobtainable if any single agency suddenly
departed from the common salary.[8]

Thus in accordance with their usual methods of salary "readjustment," a
meeting of the larger VNAs was held in consultation with the NOPHN in New
York in January 1920. After much discussion, the participants decided that
before passing judgment on the matter, it seemed prudent for each agency to

conduct an informal study to determine if they were already paying their staff a "living wage." Although unwilling to take action at this first meeting, they were able to agree that nurse's salaries should be based on a reasonable estimate of their anticipated living expenses plus enough income to save for old age or illness. In the final analysis, their studies found that many associations underpaid their staff to such a degree that saving was simply out of the question.[9]

The end result of this process was an unprecedented 52 percent increase in the average staff nurse's salary followed by a substantial increase in the size of the staff employed by these nine agencies. Having demonstrated to their own satisfaction the relationship between the nursing shortage and nurses' salaries, they took advantage of the April NOPHN convention to preach their new economic gospel to the as yet uninformed, smaller organizations. Their efforts apparently met with some success, for the 1922 survey of salaries conducted by the NOPHN documented improvement in nurses' salaries across the country.[10]

Nevertheless, within a few years many, VNAs found the demand for nursing care again exceeding their ability to attract and retain an adequate staff; often their inability to keep up with the growth of the work meant that associations had to refuse cases. Again, the issue of adequate salaries was raised, followed predictably by salary studies, raises, larger staffs, and bigger budgets.[11]

Many boards found it increasingly difficult to raise the money necessary both to pay an adequate salary to the nurses and to hire each year the additional staff necessary to keep up with the growing demand for service. It was a precarious situation, since even the most aggressive VNA only managed to collect 30 percent of their budget from patient fees, with the remainder coming from investments and contributions.[12] Thus the growing uncertainty of being able to fund an ever-increasing budget loomed over most boards—often discouraging attempts at undertaking anything new. Innovation was being replaced by their more pragmatic concern for pay patients, efficiency, and contributions.[13]

But for those nurses and board members attending the June 1924 meeting of the NOPHN, local worries were at least temporarily overshadowed by the impending financial crisis of the Instructive District Nursing Association (IDNA) of Boston. Although a dramatic situation, it must have felt all too familiar to most of the nursing leaders attending the meeting. It was a particularly ironic turn of events because, under the guidance of Beard, the IDNA had become an ideal VNA in the opinion of most observers. It offered the citizens of Boston a "generalized" neighborhood nursing program, maintained high standards of care, and had recently undergone a period of remarkable growth. As a result, while the average association provided care to twenty-one out of every one thousand residents, the IDNA cared for sixty-eight of every one thousand Bostonians. Unlike any other association, the IDNA could plausibly claim its intention of extending the services of the visiting nurse to the whole community.[14]

In order to expand the IDNA's work, seventy-five nurses had been added to the staff since the end of the war. In order to attract so many nurses, salaries had been raised on three separate occasions. As a result, the IDNA's budget increased from $150,000 in 1919 to $357,000 in 1923.[15] Operating in accordance with time-honored methods, each year Beard would present her new plans and her larger budget to the board, who would then go out and try to find the money to support it. But over the years, raising money became much more difficult.[16] Having sought the advice of some businessmen, the board decided to hire an "ad man" to help them find a more successful method of raising funds.[17] Eventually, they located such a person, a Mr. Morgan, who informed them that indeed they had made the right decision. Their budget had grown to such proportions that it could no longer be raised in what he termed "a ladylike way," meaning tag sales, annual subscriptions, and charity balls. A much more vigorous publicity campaign was now required and this was, according to Morgan, a man's job. His plan called for an advertising campaign in train stations and newspapers, hanging posters in Copley Square and the Commons, and sending girls into the hotels, department stores, and train stations to solicit contributions on an advertised date.[18]

Morgan's plans were too aggressive for the ladies on the board who decided to limit his activities to writing advertisements for the IDNA. Continuing their search for an acceptable method of fundraising, a board member was sent to Philadelphia, Providence, and New York to study their procedures. She concluded that the most successful approach to securing adequate financial support was through an educational campaign conducted by (1) a businessmen's committee, (2) local neighborhood committees, and (3) societies of young women. This more conservative approach proved more acceptable to the board and was immediately implemented.[19]

Their new methods seemed sufficient until February 1923, when it became obvious that the IDNA would end the year with a deficit of $26,000. This time, the ladies turned to the men on the board for help but found them unwilling to put in the time necessary to reorganize the work. Their response was to tell the ladies to hire a general organizational man to supervise their finances and office management and to find some way of increasing the organization's earning power.[20]

Despite their renewed efforts, by November, even Beard admitted that the question of limiting the work of IDNA was bound to come sooner or later.

The demand for service was finally reaching that point where the staff could no longer increase with it because of either lack of money or lack of properly trained nurses.[21]

Six months later, the inevitable happened. The spring appeal for funds was a great disappointment, raising $34,000 less than anticipated. Although twelve nurses had already been dismissed in April, expenses would have to be curtailed even more if the board failed to raise an additional $14,000 a month.[22] Recognizing the unavoidable outcome of such a task, Beard was asked to present a plan for "curtailment of the work" to the May 1925 meeting of the executive committee of the board. Finding any reduction less than desirable, Beard made certain her plan did not "omit the fact that local organizations [would] undoubtedly take up the work [IDNA] abandoned with probably most unfortunate results."[23]

Although the final decision to curtail the work of the Boston association by $130,000 would not be voted on by the board until the week after the June NOPHN convention, the outcome seemed obvious, and at the convention, the topic was no less avoidable.[24] Although the IDNA's rapid expansion and retrenchment seemed extreme in comparison to the experience of most VNAs, the basic issues were similar.[25]

Not surprisingly, then, the focal point of the convention was a paper and subsequent "round table discussion" presented by William Norton, secretary of the Community Fund of Detroit, on "Meeting the Demands for Community Health Work."[26] His main points included a review of available sources of revenue, a discussion of the growing competition between numerous community organizations for these funds, and the need for VNAs to rapidly convert as much of their work as possible into self-supporting enterprises. If VNAs hoped to meet the demand for their services, they had to pay the resulting bills. Public support did not just happen, he reminded his audience; it was acquired. Jargon and unexplained professional conclusions were no longer sufficient. The people who pay the bill, vote the tax, or give the gift had to first understand the problem. Second, they must be convinced that the visiting nurse was the best solution. And finally, they had to be given proof that the proposed outcome could be obtained.[27]

Although the message was not particularly innovative or even new, when coupled with the news from Boston, its impact was spectacular.[28] While some had assumed that Boston's lack of a community chest precipitated the association's financial crisis, here was the secretary of the Detroit Community Fund describing a much larger problem that could not be cured by so simple a solution as cooperative fundraising.[29] According to Mary Gardner, the message was clear; the age of discovery, aspiration, experiment, and belief without proof had been replaced by the more practical "period of the proof of the pudding." After much discussion, five points were agreed on by those present:

> First, that in all probability we cannot expect in the next ten years the same rate of financial increase we have experienced in the past ten.
> Second, that methods accepted in private life should apply to organizations—namely, no debt, and no expenditure of principle except under the rarest of conditions.
> Third, that stricter business methods should be applied to publicity and advertisement.
> Fourth, that educational work, as well as bedside nursing should be charged for and that there should be a more systematic effort to make all work self-supporting.
> Fifth, that there should be general readiness to turn over the work of private organizations to public administration.[30]

Having committed themselves to a more conservative, businesslike course of action, they all agreed that those executives who found themselves unable to balance their budgets should feel no guilt, for it was simply a sign of the times. Not only was a slowing down inevitable, but some believed a certain "curtailment" of public health nursing would occur. But this, declared Gardner, might not prove an unmixed evil, "since with it [would] come a stricter analysis and appraisal of the various types of work in light of actual results obtained."[31]

Self-analysis in terms of end results was not a new concept for visiting nursing. Dr. Lee Frankel first introduced the idea in his 1916 paper on the need for a standardized financial statement.[32] Sharing his concern, the NOPHN created the Committee on Organization and Administration with Katharine Codman, a member of the IDNA board, as chair.[33] Ironically perhaps, Mrs. Codman was the wife of Ernest Amory Codman, a Boston surgeon whose passion for evaluating medical intervention in terms of "end results" had by 1915 resulted in his forced resignation from his medical society, the loss of his teaching position at Harvard, and personal financial loss.[34] Possibly, Mrs. Codman did not share her husband's enthusiasm, for under her leadership, the committee accomplished little of substance.[35]

The first substantial analysis of public health nursing was the Goldmark Report, which after several delays was finally published in 1923.[36] In its search for an appropriate educational basis for public health nursing practice, the study examined through "discriminating observation" the successes and failures of 141 nurses and, to a lesser extent, the organization and administration of thirty-seven public health nursing organizations. The study produced no real surprises, but it did, as one reviewer noted, reaffirm what the nursing leaders had been saying for years.[37]

While Goldmark's recommendations mirrored in every respect the wishes of the visiting nurse leadership, obtaining the unanimous support of the committee for their views had proven a difficult task. Because the study was expanded in 1920 to include all nursing education, the committee had also grown—producing, from a nursing perspective, a less friendly and pliable membership.[38] The outcome was, according to Anne Strong, a group of "warring, forceful, unreconcilable individuals with all their different complexes." That they ever came to any agreement was, she concluded, "a miracle sort of like mixing oil and water."[39]

Most heartening for the visiting nurses was the committee conclusion that, despite past objections of official health agencies, best results would be achieved when the public health nurse was able to combine nursing in sickness with preventive educational measures. Consistent with the claims of visiting nurse leadership, the advantages of this approach were "repeatedly and unmistakably demonstrated." Based on this belief, the committee dismissed the idea of a nonnurse health visitor by recommending "that the teacher of hygiene in the home should possess in the first place, the fundamental education of the nurse" supplemented by a graduate course in the special problems of public health. While the committee supported the development and strengthening of university schools of nursing, their more immediate concern was the need for higher admission standards and a shorter period of higher quality training for all nurses. Finally, it recommended that a "subsidiary worker" be used in public health nursing agencies to assist the nurse with cases of mild and chronic illness.[40]

While Goldmark applauded public health nursing's "palpable achievements" and reaffirmed its future promise, her study documented numerous problems. Public health nursing's first attempt at self-analysis, while perhaps not entirely systematic, produced some dismaying findings. "Broadly speaking," the investigation found that only 47 percent of the nurses were "successful" in practice, 29 percent provided average care, and 25 percent were unsuccessful. Success was judged on the basis of personality, teaching ability, technique, social understanding, and organizational skill.[41]

In the final analysis, the committee concluded that both the responsibilities and prospects for improvement rested on the training schools and, to a lesser extent, with the agencies employing the nurse. Nursing education was, according to Winslow, chair of the committee, "an unsatisfactory compromise and its products neither good enough to be saved nor bad enough to be damned." Public health nursing's ability to successfully carry out its functions in the future could only be achieved, he suggested, through substantial educational reform.[42]

If implemented, the recommendation of the Goldmark Report would have meant that official health agencies should join with the visiting nurses to form an amalgamated organization providing both curative and preventive nursing services, the hiring of some type of ancillary worker to care for the growing number of chronically ill patients requiring home care, and "higher caliber," better-educated women entering the field of public health nursing. But by the 1924 NOPHN convention, the Goldmark Report had failed to produce any significant changes in nursing education, much less in the delivery of public health nursing services.[43]

While the Goldmark Report addressed the question of quality of care as it related to nursing education, a second major study conducted by the Committee to Study Visiting Nursing set out to examine quality of care in relation to cost. The conclusions of the committee were presented the same afternoon as the Round Table on Meeting the Demand for Community Health Work.[44]

The study was conducted and published at the expense of the Metropolitan Life Insurance Company (MLI), whose primary concern was establishing an estimate of comparative efficiency based on cost per visit.[45] Unfortunately, the committee found so little information about the most "simple facts" in the majority of agencies that their conclusions were more qualitative than quantitative. Although they could not determine what constituted the usual nursing workload or even the frequency of care in various types of cases, they did obtain some data on staff age, education, turnover, and NOPHN membership. They were able to establish that the average nurse spent 19 percent of her day in the office writing records and 77 percent of the day in the field. Forty-three percent of her time was spent in the patients' homes and 25 percent was accounted for by travel. The average nurse made nine visits a day, with the average visit lasting twenty-two minutes.[46]

On the whole, the investigators were pleased with the nursing techniques and actual patient care they observed but found that the patients' records often failed to accurately reflect the care provided. Like the Goldmark study, they found the nurses' ability to determine the family health situation, to teach prevention or even routine home nursing, and to recognize nonmedical situations affecting family and community health less than satisfactory. Thus while the nursing leadership were claiming the emphasis of public health nursing had shifted from "bedside care in its narrower sense to family health work with education as its basis," both studies documented that the practice of most public health nurses failed to conform to this ideal.[47]

Finally, because of the extreme variations in agency accounting methods, the committee found it impossible to compute the cost of a visit on any consistent basis. Instead they chose to outline a uniform system of accounting by which the standardization necessary for further comparison could be accomplished.[48]

Although the data were superficial, the study did provide the first opportunity for most public health nursing agencies to evaluate their efficiency in terms of some external criteria. But as one critical reviewer pointed out, the report provided few real "findings." It was, instead, more like a recommended plan for agency reorganization on a businesslike basis.[49] When asked to comment on the report, Frankel expressed his "tremendous gratification" with this piece of research but went on to say that this should simply be the beginning of a series of studies of visiting nursing.[50]

Frankel's wish was fulfilled. Having adopted "the modern attitude" of scientific study, visiting nurses were obsessed by self-analysis and appraisal for the remainder of the decade. They examined output to cost in terms of quality, time per visit, interval of visits, analysis of visit content, record keeping, average time expended by type of health problem, and even cost per minute. As the data accumulated, they produced estimates of "nurse power" as well as nursing progress. Ultimately, they assumed these evaluation tools would become sophisticated enough to allow comparison between various methods of work and to eventually produce service norms or generalizable standards.[51]

While public health nursing acquired a more "intelligent appreciation" of the value of self-analysis, it barely acknowledged Gardner's plea that they begin to plan intelligently for future developments by examining their work in terms of "outstanding results."[52] Neither the questions asked nor the conclusions reached deviated significantly from the earlier studies. Their focus was inward, toward issues of productivity and financial survival, rather than outward, toward end results or analysis of community need. Not unique to either visiting nurses or their organizations, these concerns were, not surprisingly, shared by the medical profession as well as the modern hospital. But unlike the modern hospital, visiting nursing's failure to look outward proved a costly mistake.[53]

In March of 1925, Frankel, whose vision was apparently not as constricted, approached the NOPHN with an offer to finance a small regional conference to discuss trends in public health work and to begin planning for the next ten years. Nurses had been the least articulate of the public health groups and were, he suggested, consequently in danger of having decisions made for them. They must consider the underlying reasons for their present activities as well as the basis for "the division of responsibility for community health work between public health nursing associations and other community health agencies, official and non-official." Ultimately, he advised, they must decide whether present trends were a satisfactory goal or if they should begin to formulate some policy for the future and work toward it. While agreeing to the conference, the executive committee approved of only a portion of Frankel's agenda. Clarification of thought was acceptable, but forming conclusions or the making of ultimata for others to follow were not seen as desirable outcomes. From the NOPHN's perspective, the only consequence, beyond discussion, that might conceivably develop was the appointment of a committee to consider the issues raised.[54]

Twelve VNAs were invited to send their "executive" and a board member to the conference, which was held in New York City in April 1925. Unlike the NOPHN, the participants were willing to put the future to a vote. But unfortunately, their analysis of the coming decade proved to be as unrealistic as the NOPHN's reaction was conservative. With two participants in opposition, it was voted that in the future, nursing in the home and prenatal and postnatal care would be done by their private agencies but subsidized with public funds, that care provided in clinics should be carried on by hospitals, and that health departments ought to limit their work, more or less, to the exercise of police powers when necessary for the preservation of the community's health.[55]

Their vote demonstrated visiting nursing's disdain for health departments' ability to deliver nursing services and their continuing belief that VNAs would eventually become the legitimate recipients of public funds. They could not understand why municipalities were willing to acknowledge their obligation to underwrite nursing care in hospitals and yet felt such care to be "superfluous" in the home. Municipal assessment of community need would, they hoped, ultimately demonstrate the wisdom of their conclusions. In the end, it would become obvious how much less expensive it was to care for patients in the home.[56]

While they privately contemplated the demise of the health department, the visiting nursing leadership publicly campaigned for amalgamation. The term *amalgamation* was used to describe those organizations that through a variety of methods combined the predominantly curative services of the voluntary nursing organization with the predominantly preventive services of the publicly funded agency to form a single public health nursing association

(PHNA). Visiting nurses supported this idea because it eliminated duplication of services, ended competitive feelings between voluntary and public nursing organizations, reunited the curative and preventive functions of the public health nurse, and better met the needs of most patients more effectively. Although a less loudly proclaimed outcome, amalgamation also assured voluntary agencies greater access to public funds and legitimated their claims that they too contributed to the public's health.[57]

Although the *PHN* ran a series of articles that the editors claimed demonstrated the trend toward amalgamation and reported the details of numerous supportive studies, little really changed.[58] Health departments never shared the visiting nurses' affinity for amalgamation, no doubt viewing any unnecessary association with curative programs as an unwise extension of their public health activities.[59] By 1931, few health departments provided bedside care and only 20 percent of all PHNAs were combined agencies.[60] Despite their lack of immediate success, the NOPHN clung to this idea as the only sensible solution to the economic problems of the voluntary associations. The NOPHN's final study of combined public health nursing agencies was conducted in 1949.[61]

While visiting nurses failed in their efforts to obtain "public funds," they did, in some communities, receive public recognition and support for their work from community chests or welfare federations. While these funds provided a degree of financial relief, they rarely allowed for much expansion or experimentation, much less any aggressive attempt to reorder the health-care system.[62]

In the absence of strong community financial support, VNAs began to accept the reality that philanthropic contributions could no longer be counted on as the basis of fiscal well-being. Likewise, having examined productivity, efficiency, budget controls, and service costs, it was equally obvious that survival required more than the practice of good business methods. Becoming more self-supporting seemed the only viable solution and this, they concluded, required giving renewed attention to the pay patient.[63]

Visiting nursing's realization that most pay patients were sick at home while few purchased the services of a nurse during illness suggested the basis for what should have proven a mutually beneficial solution. What the middle class needed was intermittent, affordable skilled nursing care, while the only care available was that provided by fulltime private-duty nurses whose fees were beyond the means of most patients. Visiting nursing's solution was nursing care sold by the hour.[64] Unfortunately, they discovered that their hourly service placed them in competition with the private-duty nurses who, as one study suggested, were already "broken in spirit, poor in purse."[65]

While realizing that an hourly service presented the most promising avenue to both survival and expansion, VNAs failed to vigorously pursue this potentially lucrative field. To succeed, they quickly discovered, this service must be made available on an appointment basis, patients must be seen by the same nurse for each visit, and a great deal of publicity was required to ensure its use by the community. Some observers suggested that in addition to these substantial organizational problems, some associations feared they might lose their philanthropic status in the eyes of their supporters.[66]

But much more important than any of the obvious constraints was the reality that hourly work was of a different "character" and tended to be more like private-duty nursing than public health nursing.[67] From the staff's perspective, hourly patients were simply too well to do and the nature of their problems too chronic. The well to do required a more leisurely approach, they discovered, and were "more talkative and less teachable." They rarely thought of helping themselves, and some even asked the nurses to perform maid services.[68] Likewise, chronic patients required simple care easily handled by someone less skilled than a nurse. While the staff realized they were filling a need, they found hourly work a burden, believing they were being asked to provide services to patients whose problems did not really require a well-trained public health nurse. Although asserting their ability to offer a service superior to that provided by the average private-duty nurse, they demonstrated little willingness to give any preference to the needs of their hourly patients over those of their other more "needy" patients.[69]

Thus in the final analysis, doing anything that made the work of the visiting nurse seem more like private-duty nursing than public health nursing rapidly dampened their enthusiasm. Not surprisingly then, while VNAs initiated hourly services, they did so in such a manner as to guarantee that they would never "encroach," in any way, on their regular services. The outcome was less than spectacular.[70]

While at home, the VNAs were discovering the difficulties of providing hourly services, at the national level, the NOPHN was acting to protect their interests from the misplaced aspirations of the other nursing organizations. While the NOPHN did not object to other nurses showing interests in the field, they did expect them to do so only under their supervision. The forum for discussion was the Joint Committee on Distribution, which was cooperatively funded in 1928 by the NOPHN, the American Nurses Association (ANA), and the National League for Nursing Education (NLNE). Through careful committee appointments, the NOPHN worked to assure the achievement of outcomes they desired. While publicly creating the image of a cooperative endeavor, in the end, the ANA chose to take no significant steps to organize hourly nursing on the behalf of private-duty nurses. The distribution of nurses within the community was, they claimed, the responsibility of the NOPHN, not theirs.[71]

Although visiting nurses claimed to have tried to meet the needs of the pay patient, some of their strongest supporters correctly criticized their efforts as superficial.[72] Even Michael Davis, who as director of the Rosenwald Fund had supported the only major study of hourly nursing, eventually reached a point of exasperation. Visiting nursing was, he declared, twenty-five years behind the hospital in its efforts to expand services among people who could pay their way. While hospitals were proud of the proportion of services rendered to pay patients, VNAs with a similar social obligation were, from his perspective, timid about it. Hourly nursing was not considered an integral part of the visiting nurses association's policy, but it was considered a secondary activity and was administered more as a concession than an opportunity. As a result, Davis concluded, it tended to be too inflexible to meet the needs, much less the demands, of the people who should utilize it.[73]

Surveys in 1927 and 1931 confirmed that hourly nursing had indeed become a lost opportunity for most VNAs.[74] Confronted by their lack of success, visiting nurses were at last forced to begin to question why. In contrast to Davis, they concluded that the failure of hourly nursing to meet the needs of patients of moderate means was probably the result of simply overestimating the need or, perhaps, their failure to offer the service in a form that met the patients' requirements or wishes. The resolution of this dilemma was left to the representatives of the NOPHN, ANA, and NLNE on the Committee on Community Nursing.[75]

Eventually, VNAs did become more self-supporting, not because of the pay patients alone, but more because of the growing number of patients whose insurance policies paid for the services of a visiting nurse during illness. By the end of the decade, most VNAs earned at best 35–45 percent of their budgets from private patients and insurance fees.[76] In contrast, by 1922, 65 percent of general hospital income came from patient fees.[77]

But by 1930, even this source of income had begun a rather dramatic decline. From an insurance company's perspective, the visiting nurse no longer seemed an economical method for preventing death. The reality was that as the care of the acutely ill increasingly became the responsibility of hospitals, the company found itself paying for the care of the chronically ill at home. From their perspective, the outcome of chronic illness was rarely determined by nursing intervention and was, as a result, considered a poor investment. Finding that while the number of visits to policyholders was declining, the cost

of the service was rapidly growing, the companies decided to terminate their
nursing program in 1953.[78]

By the end of the decade, visiting nursing had completed the agenda
established at the 1924 convention. They had tried it all: self-analysis, self-
support, lower expectations, better management, more publicity, soliciting of
public funds, and limiting spending to income actually earned. None of these
approaches was very successful, and even before the depression, the decline of
visiting nursing seemed inevitable. By 1930, too much had changed, and visiting nurses found the evolving health-care system increasingly incompatible
with their vision of the future.[79]

The social, medical, and demographic circumstances that had created
a need for large numbers of visiting nurses twenty years earlier were simply no longer of major concern to most communities. Urban death rates
were dramatically declining and infectious diseases were being replaced by
chronic, degenerative diseases as the leading causes of death. These noninfectious diseases did not have the same kind of fluctuating, dramatic, and
often frightening impact that had originally helped prompt public concern
and philanthropic support for the visiting nurse.[80] World War I and the immigration quotas initiated in 1921 and 1924 also contributed to the changing
nature of public health nursing. Fewer immigrants and second-generation
families meant the needs of the foreign-born could no longer help legitimate
the role of the nurse as the agent of Americanization.[81] Finally, the hospital
had also undergone a major transformation since the turn of the century. An
institution that once housed the destitute sick poor was becoming a center of
research and clinical application for ideas and inventions derived from science and medical technology. What is more, the number of hospital beds was
growing six times faster than the population as medical, surgical, and even
some obstetrical patients, of all classes, began to seek hospital care.[82]

Perhaps, prophesied Tucker, by the millennium, the VNA would become
the central community health organization that offered every kind of nursing
service to patients in their home. With the rising cost of hospital care, her pre-
dictions may in fact come true. But in the interim, visiting nurses have been
forced to survive for decades within communities that no longer see them as
necessary, if they know of their existence at all.[83]

II

Peacetime brought to the national level organizations that were in most regards
similar to, though often more dramatic than, those experienced by the smaller
local associations. Like the VNAs, what began as a decade of great hopes and

dreams for the American Red Cross and the NOPHN ended with retrenchment and decline.

By the end of November 1918, the Red Cross had completed its peacetime plans, having decided to make its public health nursing program "the basis and backbone of the Red Cross endeavor." Polling its membership confirmed the appeal of this idea and launched an intensive three-month effort to turn national plans into policies and procedures that could be adapted by the local chapters. By April of 1919, they were in place, and thirty-one Red Cross nurses had been sent out on the Chautauqua circuits as a "publicity stunt." Sharing their war stories, the nurses made their "pleas for a new era of health" directed by the Red Cross and financed by local communities. Money presented few immediate obstacles, since most local chapters had a residue of funds from their war efforts as well as a core of workers eager to replace their war duties with another "big cause." The "great boom," as Gardner called it, was overwhelming. Hundreds of chapters with money in hand sought the Red Cross's assistance in establishing public health nursing services—preferably overnight.[84]

In one year, the number of nurses employed by the Red Cross quadrupled from 97 to 472. Twenty percent of the thirty-seven local chapters initiated some kind of public health nursing services, leaving Nevada the only state without at least one such program.[85] Like the VNA, they found the major obstacle to implementing their plans to be a lack of qualified public health nurses. By 1920, Elizabeth Fox, director of the program, estimated a potential need for sixteen hundred more nurses and a pressing need for one thousand more nurses within the next six months. With only ten thousand public health nurses anywhere in the country, the demand, suggested Fox, had "speedily outrun" the supply.[86]

The Red Cross simply could not keep up with the local chapters' demands for more nurses. Between the fall of 1914 and summer of 1920, an average of 68 new services opened each month, and by the latter part of 1921, there were a total of 1,240 Red Cross public health nurse services employing 1,267 nurses across the country. At its peak, the Red Cross had "launched" 2,100 services. For several years, their combined overseas and home nursing programs made the Red Cross the largest single employer of nurses in the world. Some critics began to express fears that the Red Cross was overambitious and accused them of overstimulating the situation to the point that it had gotten out of hand. While at the time, Fox staunchly defended their venture, she later described those first few years as an "alarming" period when they proceeded almost out of control.[87]

When at the end of 1921 the Nursing Division was reorganized into three separate programs, Fox was, at last, able to gain a greater degree of control over the future of the Red Cross's public health nursing program. In addition, reorganization meant Fox was no longer subjected to the reign of Clara Noyes, a woman for whom Fox had less than warm feelings. Noyes, who at the time was the president of the ANA, was not a public health nurse and, therefore, in the eyes of Fox (ironically president of NOPHN), in no way prepared to tell her how to run the public health nursing activities of the Red Cross. Despite the reorganization, their rivalry continued almost as a counterpart to that of their two organizations, the ANA and the NOPHN.[88]

In an effort to increase the supply of qualified public health nurses, the Red Cross created a scholarship and loan program, which by the time it was terminated in 1929 totaled $300,000. As a result, the Red Cross made it possible for 1,176 nurses to obtain postgraduate training in public health. Since in 1919 there were only thirteen postgraduate programs with a total capacity of only 450–500 students, the Red Cross also subsidized certain of the programs, allowing them to increase their enrollment.[89]

An inadequate supply of public health nurses was not the only problem encountered by the Red Cross. The NOPHN as well as numerous departments of health and local tuberculosis associations questioned, and even disapproved of, the Red Cross interest in public health nursing. They were particularly concerned about the rapidity of the Red Cross's expansion and the seemingly competitive nature of their enterprise. Eager to create more cooperative relationships and no doubt hoping to protect their control over what they saw as their domain, the Red Cross, the NOPHN, the National Tuberculosis Association, and the Conference of State and Provincial Health Authorities created what they called cooperative working agreements in December 1919.[90]

Despite agreement at the national level upon principles, division of labor, and methods of cooperation, local Red Cross chapters still encountered hostility. Too often, critics claimed, chapters initiated public health services with insufficient funds or staff, inadequate community support, and without cooperative agreements with existing health agencies, health officers, or local physicians. National organizations that created an artificial demand for local health programs, suggested Gardner, were viewed by many longtime visiting nurse leaders as of dubious virtue. Demand, she suggested, should come from the community. Only then could programs develop slowly, fostering as they grew the community's understanding and support. Complaints also came from VNAs who believed the Red Cross was luring away their nurses in a time of nursing shortage and from local health officers who felt ignored by yet another voluntary organization. By its 1922 convention, the American Medical Association had joined the ranks of those publicly expressing hostility toward the health work of the Red Cross.[91]

As if the external fault-finding was not enough, opposition and criticism of the public health nursing program began to come from within the Red Cross. Somewhat surprisingly, Mabel Boardman, a longtime supporter of the program, publicly accused the Red Cross of "exceeding its rights and endangering its proper obligations by engaging in extensive public health and social work activities." She regarded the Red Cross as an organization for meeting emergencies and thought it was stretching the meaning of the Red Cross charter too far to think of disease as a disaster that the Red Cross must attempt to prevent. While Boardman's remarks caused a minor sensation, as with the opinions of other assailants, they were discussed and duly dismissed.[92]

While the National Red Cross reaffirmed its commitment to the public health nursing program, the local chapters' devotion was beginning to waver.[93] The same year, many chapters began to use up their war surplus funds and failed—or chose not—to find the money necessary to continue their nursing programs. As a result, 900 Red Cross nurses found themselves unemployed. For the three years between January 1921 and December 1923, Red Cross nursing programs closed at an average rate of 363 a year. By January 1924, only 804 services and 967 nurses remained, and although the rate of "withdrawal" had declined, the end was not yet in sight.[94] Simultaneously, the nature of their nursing programs was increasingly limited to bedside care as their preventive programs were taken over by official agencies whose growth was supported by the Rockefeller Foundation, the Children's Bureau, and the Sheppard-Towner Act.[95]

Not unlike the NOPHN's response to the growing difficulties of the VNAs, the Red Cross resorted to self-analysis and "remodeling." The study of their staff was completed in 1922 and resulted in what Fox described as "an airing of the family skeleton." Despite their substantial effort to maintain high educational standards, only 48 percent of the Red Cross's public health nurses had any postgraduate training and only 7 percent had completed the recommended six- to eight-month course. Most interesting to Fox was the strong correlation found between advanced preparation and exceptional performance. Given their lack of preparation, she was not surprised to find that the performance of only 9 percent of the nurses was rated as exceptional, 41 percent was considered very good, while the remaining 50 percent was good to fair. Although the findings supported the need for the Red Cross's continued investment in the education of its staff, the money made available for loans and scholarships became smaller each year until the program was discontinued in 1929.[96]

As budgets continued to contract, the number of divisional offices and field personnel were also reduced and visits to local chapters were dramatically curtailed. Managing only an annual visit meant the nursing field representative would provide little guidance, support, or supervision. Predictably, in her absence, other new programs in first aid, home hygiene, nutrition, and family services for veterans began to compete with nursing for limited chapter funds.[97]

Looking back, Fox realized their path had been "obstructed on every side by general apprehension of the Red Cross's intentions and capacities, by vigorous opposition from health authorities, by coldness and open hostility on the part of the medical profession, by the inexperience of the chapters, by lack of standards in rural nursing and by a scarcity of qualified nurses."[98] Those chapters, she concluded, too frail for their cargo, insufficiently manned, or sailing without compass or rudder were now shipwrecked and abandoned. Those six hundred chapters that had survived the storm were "battered but seaworthy" and had come into calmer waters. Like VNAs, their storm had been one of popularity and the consequent demand that had made it impossible to maintain control.[99]

III

When in 1930 Katharine Tucker, director of the NOPHN, concluded that her organization was the "symbol and expression" of what was happening in public health nursing across the country, she was no doubt saying more than she realized.[100] Ten years earlier as president, she had equally correctly announced the end of the NOPHN's "pioneer period." As a result of their wartime activities, the public health nurse and the NOPHN had for the first time been given their "true place and full recognition" as "a permanent necessity and not an incidental luxury."[101]

Surveying the newly achieved status of the public health nurse, it seemed appropriate to Tucker to suggest an equally prestigious future for the NOPHN. Clearly, there was no longer a need for propaganda or stimulating the growth of public health nursing; the demand now vastly exceeded the supply. And as Crandall insisted, the activities of the Red Cross precluded all need for further propaganda. What was left? she queried. The NOPHN must live on, she concluded, because of, not in spite of, this unprecedented growth. While others were swamped by demands and unable to consider "ways and means," the NOPHN would come to their assistance. Assuming a role similar to "consulting engineers," they would provide advice, analysis, and expert judgment. Moreover, as the clearinghouse for ideas and the forum for discussion, their focus would remain education, standards, and legislation.[102]

Not surprisingly, like the American Red Cross and many VNAs, the NOPHN's postwar program was one of expansion in budgets, staff, and programs. Since receipts from membership fees had decreased over the previous six years from 22 percent of the budget to a meager 7 percent, the NOPHN planned to again rely on "a few friends" to finance the 135 percent increase in expenses proposed for 1920.[103] The only dissenting voice in these plans was that of the new president, Edna Foley, who persistently asked the executive committee what they thought was going to happen to the work when their "few friends got interested in something else?"[104] Foley saw it as nothing short of insane to go on at their present rate and scale; it seemed rather like eating your cake before you paid for it.[105] Her views received little support within the NOPHN, especially from Crandall.[106] But Crandall's opposition was short lived, for by February, she had decided to resign, claiming the NOPHN had entered a new and markedly different period. Changes in policy were called for, and in her judgment, a new and different administration was now required. Despite Crandall's pending departure, Foley had little success convincing the others to reconsider their plans.[107]

By May, the NOPHN had acquired a substantial deficit and was forced to question the wisdom of its plans for expansion. Acting on what they claimed was competent advice, the executive committee decided against retrenchment and chose instead to develop plans for a campaign to solicit large subscribers and new members. Cutting back on services was, they concluded, "a poor selling policy." First, it would be noticed at once by the public who would have to be told how "financially hard up" the NOPHN had become. And second, it would necessitate telling the board what Foley called "the real state of affairs," information they would find, no doubt, embarrassing when going out for subscribers.[108]

Publicly, the NOPHN described itself as facing a critical year. Like many national agencies, it too was "feeling tremendously the postwar, pre-election financial situation." Without declaring the extent of their financial difficulty, they simply asked all public health nurses to help prevent the retrenchment of the NOPHN at the moment of its "greater usefulness."[109]

As had become their custom, the NOPHN turned to the Rockefeller Foundation for help in "meeting certain demands in connection with increasing their budget." The basis of their appeal was the need for a "steadying influence" in the field of public health nursing until the completion of the Goldmark Report. The guidance and support needed, they argued, could only be given by an organization, which was in every way acceptable to state departments of health, Red Cross chapters, tuberculosis associations, educational institutions, and other agencies. Its leaders, of course, believed the NOPHN was just such a body. While acknowledging the importance of the NOPHN, the foundation was unwilling to contribute to its general financial campaign.[110]

By October, the NOPHN's situation had grown so much worse that the executive committee realized they had no alternative but to make their deficit public.[111] In desperation, they hired the John Price Jones Company to manage a campaign that they were assured would result in forty thousand new members.[112] Even after ending the year with a $45,000 deficit, it still took the executive committee several more months to agree to retrenchment.[113]

By that time, Foley had had enough of what she described as the executive committee's "frequent and seemingly ineffectual meetings" and she too had resigned. Her major regret was that instead of having the opportunity to initiate some of her ideas that she thought would have been of use to public health nurses at large, she had been forced to spend all her time raising money that constantly "disappeared into a huge and yawning hole."[114] Following Foley's resignation, Fox, vice president of the NOPHN and director of the Red Cross Public Health Nursing Service, "stepped into her shoes."[115]

By April 1921, it was clear that not only had the John Price Jones campaign failed, but a second plan to secure members through their decentralized state committees of friends of public health nursing had met a similar fate. Foley's warnings had quickly become reality: individual contributions had decreased, the Rockefeller Foundation and the American Red Cross failed to renew their appropriation to the NOPHN, and several of the larger individual contributors were no longer willing to continue their support.[116]

Thus the NOPHN was forced to publicly announce its plight, first in the *PHN* and then at the 1922 convention. Fox was, no doubt, correct when she suggested that her audience at the convention was "doubtless only too painfully familiar" with similar fundraising difficulties. Nor were they surprised to hear that the NOPHN, like many other organizations, found itself unable to raise the desired budget and was being forced to retrench.[117] Even though Frances Payne Bolton once more came to their rescue by paying their debts, to remain solvent, the NOPHN was forced to reduce their annual expenses from $100,000 to $36,000.[118]

During the year, several plans for support were presented to the members, and all shared the common goal of increased lay membership as the means for ensuring financial survival. Economic reality had forced the NOPHN to realize that its future depended on lay, not nursing, membership. Nurses, they had learned, contributed "thought, professional knowledge and service," not money. If nurses had demonstrated anything beyond a shadow of a doubt it was, declared Gardner, their inability to meet the financial responsibilities of the NOPHN. Even if all the public health nurses in the country joined the NOPHN, their dues would only contribute a portion of the total budget and, as it was, only half belonged.[119]

Unlike the nurse members who were simply expected to pay dues, it was hoped that lay members who were "genuinely and permanently interested in public health nursing" would "decide on an annual contribution perhaps of fifty dollars, one hundred dollars, five hundred dollars or even one thousand dollars." In the future, the executive committee expected that one-quarter of the budget would come from the nurse members, one-half would come from lay members, and one-quarter would come from endowments, large gifts, and foundations.[120]

Characteristically, the most relentless advocate of the campaign for lay members was the NOPHN's largest contributor. But Bolton's support could no longer be obtained gratuitously. The fact was, she reminded the board, "that the responsibility for the upbuilding and protection of the public's health through the public health nurse belonged as much to the laity as to the nurse." In what one observer described as "short, lucid, throbbing sentences," Bolton explained one last time that the laity would continue to accept the financial burden for the NOPHN only if it included a share in the planning and management of the work.[121]

Recognizing the need to comply with the views of Bolton's, the NOPHN's constitution was again revised to provide "larger suffrage" for the lay membership. In an effort to forestall any nursing opposition, Fox wrote an article for the *PHN* in which she reminded all nurses that they had "no exclusive rights" to the field but must instead join with those laywomen who were their "allies in the war against disease."[122]

Despite their efforts, by 1924, the leadership of NOPHN was beginning to wonder how much longer so many national organizations could continue to exist.[123] They questioned the wisdom of the nursing community supporting three organizations and two magazines and even considered the possibility of joining with the ANA. But after a brief analysis, provoked no doubt by their continuing financial troubles, the board concluded that the NOPHN was still vitally needed. They would make yet one more "valiant effort" to raise the necessary funds.[124] Apparently motivated by the conclusions reached by those attending the Round Table Discussion "Meeting Demands with the Available Funds," the executive committee voted to mend their ways. It was, they concluded, the duty of an honest organization to live within its income, and as a result, the NOPHN announced its plans to reduce its expenditures by $10,000 and to find some way to pay off its $15,000 deficit.[125]

In an editorial, the NOPHN reminded its members that while "demands have continued to crowd upon it in seemingly undiminished numbers, . . . former props of the structure [were] no longer available." With their limited budget, their task was now one of putting off and limiting demands for service. They urged the members to consider if there was still some part of the structure of the NOPHN that should "come away or should be remodeled." If so, they should crystallize their thoughts for that purpose before coming to the 1926 convention.[126]

In the interim, the NOPHN sought a solution for its decline in the same fashion it chose for the VNAs: self-analysis. A study was initiated in October 1925 and was conducted by Gardner with "a view to recasting" the functions of the NOPHN.[127] Gardner wanted to find out what the organization was doing and what effect this work was having on the outside community.[128] After several months of internal analysis, she sought the advice of seven of the larger VNAs. As a result of their conference, Gardner discovered that although there was a perceived need for the NOPHN, most associations felt they had gotten more from the organization in the past. The present benefits seemed insubstantial. To most, the NOPHN represented a potential value, similar to investing in a "fire department or police department."[129]

At the end of six months, Gardner presented her report to the NOPHN. Concluding "that the work being done [was] good, needed, and [could] be done only by the NOPHN"; she had no radical suggestions or improvements to make.[130] In fact, she only suggested future options that had been and would continue to be under consideration for some time. Basically, she recommended that eventually the NOPHN limit its functions to community services and the part public health nurses and public health nursing organizations might and should play in such services. Under this new plan, public health nursing education would become the responsibility of the NLNE, while the ANA and the newly formed nursing section of the American Public Health Association (APHA) would assume responsibility for the distinctly professional aspects of public health nursing.[131]

Hence public health nursing was about to enter what Fox called an era of consolidation. They had for too many years held themselves aloof from the concerns of "the great profession of nursing." While in the past they could claim to be too busy with their new work, that excuse no longer existed. The nursing leadership concurred; in the future, there would inevitably be less distinction between nurses. In the opinion of both organizations, changing battlefields and new enemies required the creation of better and more stable conditions within the whole profession. Achieving this aim required a concerted effort to create one professional magazine and one professional organization with sections representing the profession's special interest. But despite their reconciliation, little of significance changed during the next twenty-five years.[132]

While becoming less aloof, the NOPHN was also growing more solvent. By 1927, they not only were, at last, out of debt but had also acquired a $5,000 surplus. Solvency was the result of a new scheme that encouraged member agencies to contribute 1 percent of their revenues to the NOPHN. While few contributed the full 1 percent requested, the number of agencies adopting the "percentage plan" increased from 51 in 1925 to 157 in 1929. The other new source of income came as the result of the NOPHN's decision to no longer provide the PHN free to members. Although the magazine still ran at a loss of $4,000–$5,000 each year, this represented a vast improvement over its past financial record. At the end of the decade, 22 percent of the NOPHN budget came from the "percentage plan," while the magazine contributed 25 percent. In contrast to these improvements, income from individual member's dues had decreased slightly from 20 percent in 1925 to 17 percent of the budget in 1929. Contributions had also declined from 57 percent to 30 percent of income during the same period.[133]

While attempting to maintain its improved financial status, the NOPHN continued its examination of the related and perplexing issue of lay membership. At the 1926 convention, lay members, apparently tired of waiting for the nurses to give them equal recognition, formally requested their own section within the NOPHN. The outcome was, of course, the appointment of a committee "to study the advisability of a lay section." After two years of meetings and the completion of a "careful study of lay interest in public health nursing," the Board and Committee Member Section was formed at the 1928 convention. A generous contribution by Bolton's brother assured the continuation of the section's work by allowing the appointment of their own full-time secretary to the staff of the NOPHN.[134]

Lay members were also given their own section—the Board Members Forum—in the PHN and work was begun on a board member manual. The same year, one of the largest and probably most prestigious of a series of institutes for board members was presented in New Haven. Two hundred delegates from ninety-eight VNAs attended the three days of meetings. The list of speakers was most impressive: Haven Emerson, Winslow, Allen Burns, Goodrich, Gardner, Anne Hanson, Tucker, George Vincent, and Fox. By 1930, the executive committee was finally ready to remove all restrictions on the voting power of lay members. This seemed safe, they concluded, because there was little likelihood of a "strictly professional" question being put to a vote.[135]

During the summer of 1929, Tucker, the new executive director of the NOPHN, and her assistant traveled across the country in an effort to get to know people and to discuss the future of the NOPHN. They found that many associations no longer felt any real need for help from NOPHN and thought merging with the ANA was a good idea. There was also a general feeling expressed by those visited that the larger VNAs controlled the NOPHN, while the smaller associations had little or no voice in matters. Many found the programs of the NOPHN abstract and academic. Finally, they felt the main interest of the NOPHN was educational, and especially the education of board members.[136] Ironically, only a few years before, it was the board members who felt equally neglected while the larger organization had concluded that it was the smaller agencies that primarily benefited from the programs of the NOPHN.[137]

Thus by the end of the decade it was no longer clear who the NOPHN was serving or how well they served any particular constituency. Like their clients, the visiting nurse and the VNAs, its future seemed much less clear than it had at the beginning of the decade. The only thing that seemed certain was that in the future the NOPHN would, as Wald put it, no longer grow like mushrooms. Perhaps, she concluded, that was just as well since "mushrooms are for trimming, but rather taxing as a whole meal."[138] The 1920s had failed to materialize into the decade of uncompromised expansion, public support, and financial security that the leaders of public health nursing had envisioned at the close of the war. Gone were the dreams of the earlier leaders, replaced during the postwar period by what the NOPHN called "constructive readjustment of programs to the support." Putting off and adjusting demand had become the new task.[139] Gone too were many of the outspoken advocates of social reform who found themselves out of step in this new world of pragmatic administration and careful economy. Beard now worked for the Rockefeller Foundation; Ellen LaMotte was in Europe writing; Lent lived in New York City where she sold antiques; Crandall, who had also left the profession, had joined the staff of a foundation; and Frankel had died.[140]

While the new leadership of the NOPHN remained confident in their vision of where things ought to go, they no longer seemed able to find the means to make it happen. On June 19, 1952, the members of NOPHN held their last meeting, voted the dissolution of their organization, and transferred its interests and resources to the NLNE. In December of the same year, their magazine, *Public Health Nursing*, ceased publication.[141]

IV

Not all public health nursing organizations spent the 1920s seeking new sources of revenue or at best learning to live within a modest budget. In contrast to the experience of most VNAs, Red Cross chapters, and the NOPHN, public health nursing within official agencies was undergoing a period of steady expansion. According to Gardner, the growth of public agencies had begun to outstrip that of their private counterparts as early as 1916.[142] By 1924, 58 percent of all public health nurses worked for official agencies, while 52 percent of all public health nursing agencies were publicly funded boards of health or education. Only in New England did voluntary public health nursing predominate over official agencies. Inevitably, the future of public health nursing would become the responsibility of official health agencies.[143]

Typically, the leadership of the NOPHN reacted to this seemingly uncontrolled growth with concern. Their misgivings were not unfounded, for, in fact, public health nursing within official health agencies was a very different proposition for one reason—the health officer. They correctly feared that these "public servants" might not choose to maintain the standards of work "as high as those solicitously upheld by voluntary organizations."[144]

Health departments were not run like the VNAs, a cooperative effort of ladies and nurses guided, of course, for the most part by the nurses. In contrast, the work of the public health nurse in the official agency reflected the policy of her organization. She was expected to "understand and respect the viewpoint of those with whom she must work, and foremost among these [was] the physician." Above all else, the nursing staff was counted on not to act in an independent role. Nursing policy, in most cases, was established by the health officers, occasionally in consultation with an advisory council or the board of health but rarely with the advice of the nurses.[145] Not surprisingly, the overriding concern of most health officers was to create policy that guaranteed that the preventive endeavors of his staff never endangered the continued cooperation or support of the medical community. High on his list of folly was the public health nurse who failed to exercise care not "to overstep the bounds of basic relationship between physician and nurse" by interfering with the established practice of medicine within the community.[146]

The leadership of the NOPHN found this situation less than acceptable for numerous reasons. First was the lack of stability that resulted when changes in city administration produced changes in health officers and ultimately changes in nursing policy. More unacceptable was the fact that the average health officer was not trained in public health work and was, from their perspective, simply an opportunistic physician looking for part-time work. Since nursing was only one of his many concerns, it neither received the attention it deserved nor was it allowed to function independently. Knowing little about public health nursing, much less its standards, the average health officer set policy and hired staff as best fit his needs. According to one critic, they were "likely to employ untrained home talent," often someone who had nursed someone in one of the "official families." These nurses were usually without public health nursing experience and were viewed by the NOPHN as unqualified to lead themselves, much less other nurses.[147]

This scenario, according to Fox, proceeds forward with the health officers leaving public health nursing to the nurse's discretion as long as there was no trouble.[148] Should a competent nurse be hired, by chance, she would encounter inertia and opposition whenever she tried to implement any aggressive plans that might disturb the status quo. Given such circumstances, Fox claimed, qualified nurses rarely accepted jobs with health departments. Such nurses were unwilling to work for organizations where their hands were tied "by official ignorance," opposition to progressive programs, and halfway measures. Thus official positions, contended Fox, tended to be filled by "inexperienced nurses or by nurses who have not made good under the high standards of voluntary organizations." The outcome was "hopeless mediocrity in public service."[149]

Fox's claim that this was the typical situation was neither consistent with the views of those trying to raise standards for health officers nor inconsistent with the findings and recommendations of the various studies conducted as the basis for creation of an "ideal health department."[150] When voluntary and official health agencies were compared, it was found that more adequate supervision was provided by voluntary agencies and that their staff was better prepared in terms of both education and experience. The nurses who ran the voluntary agencies were, on the whole, better qualified than those in public agencies and more often met the qualifications set by the NOPHN.[151]

Just as Fox claimed, the 1921 and 1924 studies of large cities conducted by the APHA and of small cities conducted by the American Child Health Association (ACHA) found that while most health officers were physicians, few had special training in public health work, less than half had previous experience in the field prior to their present appointment, and only 50–60 percent were full-time. The APHA study found that 40 percent of health officers operated alone, without oversight of a board of health or an advisory committee, while the ACHA study found this to be the case in 19 percent of the cities they studied.[152]

Claiming the maintenance of standards as one of its main purposes, the NOPHN leadership sought every opportunity to improve what from their perspective were deplorable conditions.[153] The time had come, they concluded, for the NOPHN to place much more emphasis on what was happening in official health agencies. What they needed was an arena where their concerns would be heard by health officers. This was the APHA.[154]

Winslow strongly supported this enterprise. He had "tired of listening to symposia on nursing questions arranged entirely by physicians" and thought a nursing section should be created within the APHA for directors of public health nursing programs employed by state and municipal health departments. By creating a "most admirable forum" for discussion, the effects of this section on the status of nurses in public health work would be far-reaching. Such a section, he believed, would never become a dangerous rival to the NOPHN, since these women would belong to both organizations, while "the great body of staff nurses" would go to the NOPHN's meetings. While Winslow, Henry Vaughan of Detroit, and Charles Hastings of Toronto advocated this move, others who "consider the nurse merely an instrument to be used by others for their ends" formed the opposition. While Winslow assured the NOPHN that no section would be created without their approval, he urged their support.[155]

While lauding his motives, the NOPHN disagreed with his methods. They too were eager to create the opportunity for public health nursing leaders to proceed with the education of health officers, but they feared that if given their own section, they would instead become isolated and unable to interact with the health officers. Of course, they also saw no need to create yet another nursing organization. Instead, they proposed the appointment of nurses to the governing council of the APHA and that they "mingle more in the meetings" of the existing sections.[156]

Winslow presented the views of the NOPHN to the executive council of the APHA, but unswayed, they voted to organize a provisional section on public health nursing "if requested by the NOPHN."[157] The section had its debut at the 1922 convention with Fox, president of the NOPHN, elected chair of what she called "our baby section." The next year, the public health nursing section was appointed as a regular section of the APHA and three of its members were elected to the governing council.[158]

Their past experiences in similar NOPHN activities proved an adequate training program for nursing's APHA undertakings. Through joint sessions, committee appointments, and cooperative surveys they gained access to the health officers. Although their numbers remained small, they rapidly gained support for their views within the APHA.[159]

In an effort to re-create the "visiting nurse association ideal" within health departments, the NOPHN leadership chose the idea of a lay advisory committee on public health nursing as their solution. This remedy created a lay body responsible for policy, program control, and appointment of the nursing staff. Having created a buffer between the nurses and the health officer, it was apparently assumed that, as in the voluntary agency, the nurses would be able to gain control of nursing matters. Although this idea gained the support of the APHA, the number of lay committees actually created remained rather small.[160]

Even though APHA reports and surveys rapidly incorporated standards and proposals acceptable to the NOPHN, creation of the ideal health department proceeded with much less haste. From the NOPHN's perspective, little had happened to solve the predictable conflicts that existed between the well-qualified public health nurse and the underprepared health officer. By 1927, although a number of cities were carrying out some part of the plan for an ideal health department, there was no instance where a city had adopted the entire plan. Although the influence of the NOPHN within the APHA endured, it was unclear how much influence the APHA had on the activities of most health departments.[161]

No matter what the eventual outcome, the fact remained that health department nurses now had their own organization within which they could address issues peculiar to their specific institutional location. It seemed obvious that eventually these nurses would tire in their efforts to fulfill commitments to both the APHA and the NOPHN, let alone to the ANA or the NLNE. When that time came they would, no doubt, choose the APHA.

V

At the end of the decade, public health nursing paused to consider its past and plan for its future. It was a critical time, and although the depression had not yet markedly changed the organization or practice of public health nursing, some modifications seemed unavoidable.[162] Thus in 1931, at the edge of inevitable transformation, the NOPHN undertook two major projects: a survey of public health nursing administration and practice, supported by the Commonwealth Fund, and a census of public health nursing in the United States.[163] In their own words, they wanted to know what variations existed in public health nursing and, more specifically, whether they were "natural and admissible, simply representing differences of adaptation to local situations" or "divergences from fundamental principles and accepted practices." Variation, in this instance, presumably meant deviation from the views and aspirations of the visiting nurse and her organization, the NOPHN.[164]

The fundamental issue remained to define public health nursing. That such a question could still be a relevant issue after fifty years of organized activity simply indicated, explained one nursing author, the lack of unity within the field itself. It reminded her of "the three blind men who went to see the elephant and who after exploring respectively the trunk, legs and tusks of the animal, went away to argue intermittently over their partially correct, but erroneous, individual concepts." The elephant, being dumb, she explained, could not insist upon being "seen" in his entirety.[165] The NOPHN had no intention of allowing public health nurses to continue to act as dumbly as the elephant. Through their new study, all would at last "see" the field in its entirety. Unfortunately, they probably saw more than they desired.[166]

In his foreword to the survey, Farrand congratulated the NOPHN for undertaking their study with such "refreshing candor." Self-scrutiny is always much more productive of results, he suggested, when not clouded by complacency or self-interest, and "anyone who reads these chapters will be struck by the frank admissions of shortcomings as well as by the recognition of opportunity and of objectives not yet attained."[167] In other words, the results were, as one commentary suggested, not wholly flattering.[168]

The survey found that the work of the nurse in health departments and boards of education was confined to preventive and educational programs for infants, pregnant women, schoolchildren, and patients with communicable diseases. Almost no bedside care was provided by these agencies. Health departments rarely collected fees for services provided, and although they claimed their concern was the whole community, in most cases the work was limited almost entirely to the poor.[169]

Despite the efforts of the APHA and the NOPHN, the survey found no instance of a lay board being appointed to advise the nursing service. Nursing remained under the control of health officers or superintendents of education who not only appointed the director of nursing but frequently chose the whole staff. Agency policy, programs, and management were activities conducted preferably in the absence of the nursing staff.[170]

In comparison to these "official agencies," the VNAs, or PHNAs as the study chose to identify them, were very different organizations and undertook a very different task. PHNAs were nursing organizations managed by nurses and supported by boards whose members were predominantly affluent women. In these agencies, bedside sick nursing and prenatal care constituted their major activities. Despite their often stated interest in extending their services to the whole community, their clients remained the poor. The survey concluded that the services of these nurses were being neither used by patients who could pay for their care nor effectively publicized by the agencies.[171]

Furthermore, although agency policy maintained that family teaching was an important part of the nurses' work, neither instruction in prevention nor family instruction in the care of the sick was found to be an integral part of the nursing care provided. Admitting that the distinction was somewhat arbitrary, the investigators suggested that PHNAs' failure to provide preventive and educational services suggested that they dealt with and thought in terms of individuals, not the whole community. Obviously, such conclusions made it increasingly difficult to claim that visiting nurses were really public health nurses.[172]

While all private and public agencies surveyed envisioned themselves as an integral part of their communities' health-care systems, most simply operated in isolation. In general, relationships, when they existed, with other social and health organizations were at best casual and haphazard. Public health nursing was administered on an agency basis, not a community basis, and in general, few steps had been taken to establish working relationships or even divisions of responsibility in program or field activities. In many communities, this informal state of affairs permitted the continued presence of both gaps and duplication in services.[173]

But most shocking was the finding that the services that public health nurses performed least well were those that were supposedly the distinctive feature of their work—health education and supervision. Astonishingly, all public health nurses in all types of agencies were poor teachers. For those who believed that the greatest asset of the public health nurse was her ability to teach health, this finding, suggested one review of the study, came as a "severe blow." Apparently, concluded the same reviewer, public health nurses had entrée to homes but did not know how to make the most of the situation.[174]

Although public health nursing found the survey results disconcerting, these results confirmed what the NOPHN had contended for years. Nurses were trained to care for the sick, not the well. Apparently, they did best those services for which they were the most prepared. Where there was adequate supervision or when the staff had taken postgraduate courses in public health, it was reflected in the nurse's superior performance. Unfortunately, those factors enhancing the nurse's abilities as the teacher of health were more often the exception than the rule.[175]

While health education and supervision were what public health nurses did least well, the 1931 census confirmed that these were services they were most often employed to perform. Ninety-four percent of the growth in the number of agencies and 72 percent of the growth in the number of public health nurses since 1924 had occurred in official organizations, either boards of health or education.[176]

In contrast to the growing numbers of official agencies, the census was only able to identify 464 VNAs, 255 Red Cross nursing services, and seventy-one "amalgamated" organizations. While nearly all voluntary organizations were found along the eastern seacoast, public health nursing in official agencies had moved steadily westward. Thus it was not surprising to find that in 1931, most public health nurses (61 percent) and most public health nursing agencies (63 percent) were under official auspices.[177]

Hence while the number of new privately funded agencies declined, the number of local and state boards of health and education employing public health nurses increased. In these publicly funded jobs, the nurses found support for their traditional concerns—infectious diseases and health education for the poor. Even with such jobs opening to them, however, public health nurses could not maintain the central place within the health-care system that had once, if briefly, been theirs. As medical interest shifted away from problems of infection and public interest in the health of the poor declined, the concerns of public health nurses became less and less widely shared.

In "the long view of history, the grey clad nurse with the cross on her arm—climbing the stairs of the city tenement . . . may perhaps prove the symbolic figure of the century in which the results of a new science of healing were applied in a new and universal fashion to promote the well-being of mankind."[1] This is how C-E. A. Winslow thought the nurses of his time would be remembered. In retrospect, his optimistic picture appears to have been little more than wishful thinking.

Yet at the turn of the century, the future seemed to hold great promise for public health nursing. To the public and voluntary agencies who sought their services, these nurses seemed to be an economical and appropriate way to help the poor. Within a decade, the public health nurses' role had expanded to include a variety of preventive services not only for those suffering from such infectious diseases as tuberculosis but also for mothers, babies, schoolchildren, and industrial workers.

But as the number and variety of organizations hiring these nurses increased, the future direction of this new field seemed to be evolving beyond the control of its newly emerging leadership. As a result of the peculiar aims of these various agencies, bedside care of the sick was separated from the preventive aspects of the public health nurses' role. Increasingly over the years, public health nurses who were employed by visiting nurse associations (VNAs) cared for the sick at home while those working for boards of education or health were expected to simply be the teachers of prevention.

Despite these organizational realities, the leadership clung to their ideal of the public health nurse as the "community mother—the trained and scientific representative of the good neighbor," as Winslow had once described.[2] But even with organized nursing efforts to re-create an institutional framework that allowed public health nurses to give both preventive and curative care, such a role remained more a universal nursing ideal than an obtainable reality.

In the interim, the number of agencies, both voluntary and public, hiring these nurses continued to grow. By the time the National Organization for Public Health Nursing (NOPHN) and the American Red Cross Rural Nursing Service were both created in 1912, public health nurses felt confident that they had at last the opportunity to promote and establish their field throughout the country. While World War I temporarily delayed their plans, it also created new opportunity for all public health nursing organizations. With the end of the war, public health nursing's leaders looked forward to a promising future. Indeed, what followed was a period of rapid expansion, ironically followed by declining income, deficits, and contracting budgets.

Examined from any perspective, the circumstances that had created the need for these nurses twenty years before no longer existed. With fewer immigrants, declining death rates from infectious diseases, and the growing centrality of the hospital by the late 1920s, public health nurses and their organizations found themselves increasingly inconsequential. Within this new reality, VNAs as well as the NOPHN found their once-clear purpose and vision had become increasingly elusive and financial support was becoming difficult to obtain. While various methods of securing support were attempted, none proved particularly successful.

Simultaneously, the number of local and state boards of health and education employing public health nurses was increasing. But even as the preventers of infectious diseases and the teachers of health, public health nurses could not hold the central place within the health-care system that had once, albeit briefly, been theirs. As medical interest shifted away from problems of infections, and public interest in the health of the poor declined, the concerns of these public health nurses became less and less widely shared.

Thus turn-of-the-century America witnessed a special moment in the history of public health nursing when the trained nurse seemed the perfect solution to a set of complex and interrelated problems. Indeed, not only did public health nursing have considerable symbolic and practical appeal; it also offered nurses an irresistible combination—economic security and professional independence.

Developing under the aegis of a variety of disparate and different private and public agencies, however, public health nursing never generated the kinds of structures that might have enabled it to establish itself as a cohesive, recognized, and powerful group within the health-care system. Although nurses did help bring about some changes within the domain of public health, this field's development was determined predominantly by factors beyond the control of organized nursing.

Within the fee-for-service hospital-based system of medical care that has become increasingly entrenched since the 1920s, the work of the public health nurse has continued to decline in significance. During the optimistic years before World War I, it would have been difficult to predict that the public health nurse would play such a marginal role. And yet, in retrospect, it is depressingly clear that the earlier growth and promise of public health nursing was little more than a false dawn.

Acknowledgments

There are many reasons I went to nursing school, but the most important of all was my mother, Ruth Pauline Zike Buhler. Mother was born in 1910 in a very small town in Indiana. The youngest of three daughters, she was, no doubt, the one most eager to leave the country—and the family farm. Graduating valedictorian of her high school class, she had no problem being accepted at Ball State Teachers College where she was, I believe, a home economics major.

Unfortunately, when her sister became ill with tuberculosis, there was no longer enough money for her to finish college. Determined not to return home, mother decided to go to nursing school, where she would receive room, board, and training in exchange for her work. Shortly thereafter, her sister died and she returned to college, but this time she found that in comparison to the hospital, the world of the home economist was hopelessly boring. Thus her subsequent return to nursing was out of interest rather than necessity. It was also a choice not wholeheartedly supported, I might add, by her family.

My mother loved nursing; it was exciting, challenging, and fulfilling to her. As a little girl, I was often entertained by her wonderful nurse stories. She used to tell me with great pride how she made up note cards to review while picking up sheets from the linen closet; she explained that this method was necessary because there was little other time in her twelve hour day of floor duty for studying. There were equally intriguing stories of her life in the nurses' home both as a pupil nurse and later as one of the first "floor nurses" hired at her hospital in the 1930s. From her perspective, her most exciting years were spent working in the operating room, which I now realize was indeed a marvelous place in the 1930s. Finally, she told me of the great honor she felt when she became one of the first members of nursing's newly formed honorary society, Sigma Theta Tau. Mother's story is, I now know, typical of her generation of nurses.

In the 1960s, when I decided to go to nursing school, my family, not surprisingly, chose a five-year baccalaureate program. Once immersed in this new culture of collegiate education, I discovered, much to my shock, the "true" nature of mother's world of nursing. To my teachers, struggling to create a better world for nursing, my mother's diploma school was an oppressive remnant of the past they sought to destroy. Even worse, her beloved operating room was a place where only technicians, not professional nurses, worked. While their views were directed toward creating institutional change, I could not help but personalize the meaning of their reform program. Working to join the ranks of these professional nurses, I dismissed my mother's values, for I had no historical context against which to understand their relevance.

This rather lengthy story is my acknowledgment that, at last, I can again enjoy and applaud my mother's nursing stories. For this, I am particularly indebted to my dear friend and fellow historian of nursing Susan Reverby. It has been through her work that I and other nurses have, thankfully, gained a more useful perspective on nursing's past. Her faithful support through the years of my study has been equally wonderful—often going considerably beyond what anyone should ask even of a member of one's dissertation committee.

I am especially grateful to Charles Rosenberg, who first suggested I undertake this study and who has read my first attempts at writing history with both patience and care. I would also like to thank the third member of my committee, Joan Lynaugh, for her invaluable assistance as both a colleague and a historian. Finally, I wish to express special gratitude to my teacher and mentor Carolyn Williams, without whose faith and encouragement, since the 1960s, none of this would have been imaginable.

Of course, this study would not have been possible without the help of the staff at the various archives and visiting nurse associations who made their resources available to me. Financially, support from the following agencies made this research possible: the American Nurses' Foundation, Nurses' Educational Funds Inc.; the Division of Nursing, Department of Health and Human Services; and the Francis C. Wood Institute for the History of Medicine, the College of Physicians of Philadelphia. I am also indebted to Ellen Fuller, director of the Center for Nursing Research, University of Pennsylvania School of Nursing. I would particularly like to thank everyone at the College of Physicians of Philadelphia, where I completed this study as a Wood Fellow. While cloistered at this historic institution I was encouraged on through the last months of revisions by Diana Long Hall and Janet Golden.

At last, to my few family, friends, and pets who have survived this study, I would like to express my special appreciation, for I have asked them to endure more than I like to admit. Over too many years, they have somehow shown consistent enthusiasm, tolerated my endless worries, and read hundreds of pages about a fundamentally foreign subject. I simply would have never finished without their love and caring. Thanks, in addition, to the cats who willingly sat without prejudice on anything I wrote and to the dogs. And finally, while I am indebted to many, I would like to express special gratitude to my parents, John and Ruth Buhler; my brother, John; my boys, Jonathan and David; and last but not least, Maurie Kerrigan.

Notes

Foreword

1 Allan M. Brandt and Martha Gardner, "Antagonism and Accommodation: Interpreting the Relationship between Public Health and Medicine in the United States during the 20th Century," *American Journal of Public Health (AJPH)* 90 (May 2000): 707–715.

2 Ibid., 709–710.

3 Ibid., 707–715.

4 Bradley Sawyer and Daniel McDermott, "How Does the Quality of the U.S. Healthcare System Compare to Other Countries?," Health System Tracker, accessed August 2, 2019, https://www.healthsystemtracker.org/chart-collection/quality-u-s-healthcare-system-compare-countries/#item-start.

5 Quoted in John B. McKinlay, "A Case for Focusing Upstream: The Political Economy of Illness," in *The Sociology of Health and Illness: Critical Perspectives*, ed. Peter Conrad and Rochelle Kern, 2nd ed. (New York: Sage, 1986), 484–498. I (Susan Reverby) was a student of Zola's for a year in the late 1970s and heard him use this story many times.

6 There were attempts at demonstration projects—small, defined projects that were efforts to find sustainable models. See, for example, Patricia D'Antonio, *Nursing with a Message: Public Health Demonstration Projects in New York City* (New Brunswick, N.J.: Rutgers University Press, 2017).

7 Karen Buhler-Wilkerson, *Nursing and the Public's Health: An Anthology of Sources* (New York: Garland, 1989) and *No Place like Home* (Baltimore, Md.: Johns Hopkins University Press, 2003).

8 See Karen Kruse Thomas, *Health and Humanity: A History of the Johns Hopkins Bloomberg School of Public Health, 1935–1985* (Baltimore, Md.: Johns Hopkins University Press, 2016).

9 Nancy Tomes, *Remaking the American Patient: How Madison Avenue and American Medicine Turned Patients into Consumers* (Raleigh: University of North Carolina Press, 2019).

10 The Inland Steel case of 1948 granted unions the ability to include fringe benefits (health insurance) as part of their negotiable wage. See Rosemary Stevens, *In Sickness and in Wealth: American Hospitals in the 20th Century* (New York: Basic Books, 1989).

11 Susan L. Smith, *Sick and Tired of Being Sick and Tired: Black Women's Health Activism in America, 1890–1950* (Philadelphia: University of Pennsylvania Press, 1995). See also Sandra Lewenson, "Hidden and Forgotten: Being Black in the American Red Cross Town and Country Nursing Service, 1912–1948," *Nursing History Review* 27 (2019): 15–28.

12 Community health, population health, and public health are sometimes used interchangeably and have some of the same goals and strategies. All three address prevention, geographic or regional groups, communities, or groups of people identified to be at risk. Purists might say that public health and population health focus on identifying risk factors related to health and disease and policy changes, while

community health focuses on how to alleviate the risk factors. See "What Is Public Health?," CDC Foundation, accessed August 12, 2019, https://www.cdcfoundation.org/what-public-health.

13 Lillian B. Rubin, "Maximum Feasible Participation: The Origins, Implications, and Present Status," *Annals of the American Academy of Political and Social Science* 385 (1969): 21. *Welfare colonialism* was the term used by Rubin to describe welfare policy made by those other than the recipients of welfare.

14 Quote from Des Callen and Oli Fein, "NENA: Community Control in a Bind," *Health/PAC Bulletin* (June 1972): 4; see also Alice Sardell, *The U.S. Experiment in Social Medicine: The Community Health Center Program, 1965–1986* (Pittsburgh: University of Pittsburgh Press, 1988); Thomas J. Ward Jr., *Out in the Rural: A Mississippi Health Center and Its War on Poverty* (New York: Oxford University Press, 2016); and Merlin Chowkwanyun, "The War on Poverty's Health Legacy: What It Was and Why It Matters," *Health Affairs* 37 (January 2018): 47–53.

15 An exception would be Julie Fairman, "'We Went to Mississippi': Nurses and Civil Rights Activism of the Mid-1960s" (lecture, 2018 Fielding H. Garrison Lecture, American Association for the History of Medicine, Los Angeles, Calif., 2018).

16 For example, see Alondra Nelson, *Body and Soul: The Black Panther Party and the Fight against Medical Discrimination* (Minneapolis: University of Minnesota Press, 2013). The Black Panthers still operate community health centers in several U.S. cities; Barbra Mann Wall, "Catholic Nursing Sisters and Brothers and Racial Justice in Mid-20th-Century America," *Advances in Nursing Science* 32 (April–June 2009): e81–93, https://doi.org/10.1097/ANS.0b013e3181a3d741.

17 Kim Phillips-Fein, *Fear City: New York's Fiscal Crisis and the Rise of Austerity Politics* (New York: Metropolitan, 2017); and James O'Connor, *The Fiscal Crisis of the State* (New York: St. Martin's, 1973).

18 "Global," Association of Nurses in AIDS Care, accessed August 7, 2019, https://www.nursesinaidscare.org/i4a/pages/index.cfm?pageID=4708.

19 "Core Functions of Public Health," Centers for Disease Control and Prevention, 2015, https://www.cdc.gov/nceh/ehs/ephli/core_ess.htm, as cited by Marie Truglio-Landrigan and Sandra Lewenson in their book *Public Health Nursing: Practicing Population-Based Care*, 3rd ed. (New York: Jones and Bartlett, 2017).

20 Anna Clark, *The Poisoned City: Flint's Water and the American Urban Tragedy* (New York: Metropolitan, 2018).

21 Michelle Alexander and Cornell West, *The New Jim Crow: Mass Incarceration in the Age of Colorblindness* (New York: New Press, 2012).

22 Paul R. Epstein, *Changing Planet, Changing Health: How the Climate Crisis Threatens Our Health and What We Can Do about It* (Berkeley: University of California Press, 2011).

23 See, for example, *For the Public's Health: Investigating in a Healthier Future* (Washington, D.C.: National Academy of Medicine, 2012); and Karen B. DeSalvo et al., "Public Health 3.0: A Call to Action for Public Health to Meet the Challenges of the 21st Century" (discussion paper; Washington, D.C.: National Academy of Medicine, 2017), https://nam.edu/public-health-3-0-call-action-public-health-meet-challenges-21st-century/.

24 "Social Determinants of Health," U.S. Department of Health and Human Services, Healthy People 2020, 2020 Topics and Objectives, accessed June 8, 2020, https://www.healthypeople.gov/2020/topics-objectives/topic/social-determinants-of-health.

25 Ibid.; "Core Functions," Centers for Disease Control and Prevention.

26 D'Antonio, *Nursing with a Message.*

27 Theodore Brown and Elizabeth Fee, "Social Movements in Health," *Annual Review in Public Health* 35 (2014): 385.

28 See Susan M. Reverby, *Co-conspirator for Justice: The Revolutionary Journey of Dr. Alan Berkman* (Chapel Hill: University of North Carolina Press, 2020).

29 "Medicare for All," National Nurses United, accessed August 15, 2019, https://www.nationalnursesunited.org/medicare-for-all.

30 Thanks to the Public Health Nurse Leadership Group, who allowed us to participate on their biweekly call, January 10, 2019, where they discussed the issues confronting public health nurses and their work today. See also the Robert Wood Johnson Foundation Public Health Leaders Program, Campaign for Action, accessed September 15, 2019, https://campaignforaction.org/our-network/grantee-and-award-programs/public-health-nurse-leaders/.

31 Karen Buhler-Wilkerson, *False Dawn: The Rise and Decline of Public Health Nursing, 1900–1930* (New York: Garland, 1989), xiii.

Preface

1 Committee for the Study of the Future of Public Health, Institute of Medicine, *The Future of Public Health* (Washington, D.C.: National Academy Press, 1988).

2 See, for example, Allan Brandt, *No Magic Bullet: A Social History of Venereal Disease in the United States since 1980* (New York: Oxford University Press, 1987); Elizabeth Fee, *Disease and Discovery: A History of the Johns Hopkins School of Hygiene and Public Health 1916–1939* (Baltimore, Md.: Johns Hopkins University Press, 1987); Barbara Rosenkrantz, *Public Health and the State, 1842–1936* (Cambridge, Mass.: Harvard University Press, 1972); and Judith Leavitt, *The Healthiest City: Milwaukee and the Politics of Health Reform* (Princeton: Princeton University Press, 1982).

3 Shirley Ann Williams is quoted from her foreword to Zora Neale Hurston, *Their Eyes Were Watching God* (Urbana: University of Illinois Press, 1978), vii–viii.

Chapter 1 — Trained Nurses for the Sick Poor

1 Annie Brainard, *The Evolution of Public Health Nursing* (Philadelphia: W. B. Saunders, 1922), 196, 203–249.

2 These reactions to the effects of industrialization, urbanization, and immigration are described in Paul Boyer, *Urban Masses and Moral Order in America* (Cambridge, Mass.: Harvard University Press, 1978), 3–21, 123–190. See also Walter Trattner, *From Poor Law to Welfare State* (New York: Free Press, 1974); Roy Lubove, *The Professional Altruist* (New York: Atheneum, 1977); and Robert Wiebe, *The Search for Order: 1877–1920* (New York: Hill and Wang, 1967).

3 Boyer, *Urban Masses*, 143–161.

4 Ibid.

5 Judith Walzer Leavitt and Ronald Numbers, "Sickness and Health in America: An Overview," in *Sickness and Health in America*, ed. Judith Leavitt and Ronald Numbers (Madison: University of Wisconsin Press, 1978), 3–10; and Gretchen Condran and Rose Cheney, "Mortality Trends in Philadelphia: Age- and Cause-Specific Death Rates, 1870–1930" (paper presentation, Annual Meeting of the Population Association of America, Denver, Colo., 1980).

6 For a discussion of this idea, see John Duffy, "Social Impact of Disease in the Late 19th Century," in *Sickness and Health in America*, 395–402. This view of these

hazards to society can be seen in Mabel Jacques, "Home Occupation in Families of Consumptives and Possible Dangers to the Public," *Transactions of International Conference on Tuberculosis* 3 (1908): 564–569; and Rosalind Shawe, *Notes for Visiting Nurses* (Philadelphia: P. B. Lakiston Son, 1893), 10.

7   For most of the nineteenth century, hospitals were charitable institutions where only the most destitute sought care; by the end of the century, they had begun a transformation that would ultimately make them a center of scientific medicine sought out by all classes. For a discussion of this transformation, see Charles Rosenberg, "Inward Vision and Outward Glance: The Shaping of the American Hospital, 1880–1914," *Bulletin of the History of Medicine* 53 (Fall 1979): 346–391; David Rosner, *A Once Charitable Enterprise: Hospitals and Health Care in Brooklyn and New York, 1885–1915* (Cambridge: Cambridge University Press, 1982); and Morris Vogel, *The Invention of the Modern Hospital, Boston 1970–1930* (Chicago: University of Chicago Press, 1980). For a discussion of dispensary care, see Charles Rosenberg, "Social Class and Medical Care in 19th Century America: The Rise and Fall of the Dispensary," *Journal of the History of Medicine and Allied Sciences* 29 (January 1974): 32–54.

8   Brainard, *Evolution*, 193–249.

9   Ibid., 211; Harriet Fulmer, "History of Visiting Nurse Work in America," *American Journal of Nursing (AJN)* 2 (March 1902): 412; Lillian Wald, *House on Henry Street* (New York: H. Holt, 1915), 152–153; Mabel Jacques, *District Nursing* (New York: Macmillan, 1911), 1–12; and Mary Beard, "Home Nursing," *Public Health Nurse Quarterly (PHNQ)* 7 (January 1915): 44–47.

10 Rathbone's ideas about constructive systems of relief were essentially the same as those of the Charity Organization Movement in America. See Boyer, *Urban Masses*, 143–161. For an extensive discussion of the origins of district nursing in England, see Brainard, *Evolution*, 103–111.

11 Brainard, *Evolution*; and William Rathbone, *Sketch of the History and Progress of District Nursing* (London: Macmillan, 1890), 15–18.

12 Rathbone, *Sketch*, 18.

13 Brainard, *Evolution*, 111–113; and Rathbone, *Sketch*, 19–24.

14 Rathbone reportedly referred to Nightingale as his "beloved chief" in these matters. Edward Cook, *The Life of Florence Nightingale* (London: Macmillan, 1913), 2:125. Nightingale wrote both the introduction and notes for the Committee of Home and Training School's publication *Organization of Nursing in a Large Town* (Liverpool: A. Holden, 1865) and also Florence Nightingale, "Suggestions for Improving the Nursing Service of Hospitals and on Methods of Training Nurses for the Sick Poor" (August 1874). This paper is mentioned by Cook, *Life of Nightingale*, 253, 449.

15 These ideas first appeared in the *Times* on April 14, 1876, and were later published as a pamphlet, which can be found in Lucy Seymer's *Selected Writings of Florence Nightingale* (New York: Macmillan, 1954), 310–318. Nightingale also wrote the introduction to Rathbone's *Sketch*, ix–xxii.

16 Brainard, *Evolution*, 117–120; and Rathbone, *Sketch*, 24–26.

17 Brainard, *Evolution*, 143–146; and Rathbone, *Sketch*, 45–50. Lee, according to Dock, was considered the most highly trained nurse of her day. After training at St. Thomas's, she completed postgraduate courses in Berlin, Dresden, and Kaiserswerth; was a surgical sister at Kings College Hospital; and then made a tour of inspection through the hospitals of Holland and Denmark, after which she was able to gain entrance for training in the Hotel-Dieu, Lariboisiere, and Enfant Jesus

hospitals of Paris and later served under the Sisters of Charity of St. Vincent de Paul in two military hospitals. M. Adelaide Nutting and Lavinia Dock, *A History of Nursing* (New York: G. P. Putnam's Sons, 1907), 2:298–299.

18 Brainard, *Evolution*, 146–155. Lee, who had married in 1879, becoming Mrs. Dacre Craven, shared her findings and recommendations in this country at the International Congress of Charities, Correction and Philanthropy, which met in Chicago in 1893. Her paper is included in John S. Billings and Henry M. Hurd, eds., *Hospitals, Dispensaries and Nursing: Papers and Discussions in the International Congress of Charities, Correction and Philanthropy, Section III, Chicago, June 12–17, 1893* (Baltimore, Md.: Johns Hopkins University Press, 1894), 547–554.

19 Billings and Hurd, *Hospitals, Dispensaries and Nursing*, 549–551. For the subsequent expansion of these ideas, see Mrs. Dacre Craven, *A Guide to District Nurses* (London: Macmillan, 1889), 1–9. See also Rathbone, *Sketch*, 49–60.

20 Brainard, *Evolution*, 156–157, 128–129. Nightingale expressed her support for the idea of a nurses' home in her 1876 letter to the *Times*, which was her effort to raise funds to support the implementation of Lee's ideas through the founding of the Metropolitan and National Nursing Association. Seymour, *Selected Writings*, 310–318.

21 Nightingale's much-quoted response to this idea was, "I don't believe you will find it will answer, but try it—try it for a year." Brainard, *Evolution*, 158. Nightingale would write a year later, "As to your success—what is not your success!" Craven claims that Nightingale saw her as the "genius of nursing." Craven in *Hospitals, Dispensaries and Nursing*, 550. For the full quote, see either Craven in *Hospitals, Dispensaries and Nursing*, 549–550; or Brainard, *Evolution*, 165–166.

22 Brainard, *Evolution*, 166. Craven in *Hospitals, Dispensaries and Nursing*, 547–554. Craven's book on district nursing became the standard text used by many training schools in the century. See Ellen Lagemann, *A Generation of Women: Education in the Lives of Progressive Reformers* (Cambridge, Mass.: Harvard University Press, 1979), 68, 72. Craven's appearance at the 1893 World's Fair and her paper on district nursing introduced her ideas to an even larger American audience.

23 Brainard, *Evolution*, 166–179, provides a description of some of Craven's activities. Standard training was a minimum of one year in the hospital followed by a minimum of six months' training in district work. In actuality, the majority of the Queen's nurses had between two and four years of hospital experience, and many were certified midwives. For details related to training and the development of the institute, see the paper presented at the 1893 World's Fair by Amy Hughes, "The Origins and Present Work of Queen Victoria's Jubilee Institute for Nurses," in *Hospitals, Dispensaries and Nursing*, 331–539. Hughes was the honorary chair of the nursing subsection. Rathbone, *Sketch*, 116–122. In 1892, there were, according to Hughes, fifty-two affiliated associations in England, thirty-six in Scotland, six in Ireland, and seven in Wales. See Amy Hughes, "The Rise of District Nursing in England," *Charities and the Commons* 16 (April 1906): 13–16. An affiliated national system, the Country Nursing Association, was developed in rural communities. From the perspective of many rural communities, this alternative system was a great success—although seen by some nursing leaders as an unnecessary compromise. While the Country Nursing Association, affiliated with the Queen's Institute, was receiving supervision and guidance from the Queen's nurses, opposition arose from the frequent reliance of many small communities on services of the less well-trained and less expensive village or cottage nurses. The English

apparently had much less trouble with this "compromise" than did their American critics. See Brainard, *Evolution*, 177. According to Amy Hughes, "There are certain centers where the village nurse is the right woman in the right place." Hughes had followed in the footsteps of Craven as superintendent of the Metropolitan and National Nursing Association, which had become one of the major training centers of the Queen's Institute. Her positive judgments are in strong contrast to Dock, who saw these nurses as an assault to the standards established by Nightingale. They were cheap nurses, she contended: "Call them what one will, the cottage nurses are not nurses." No lasting good would come, she contended, from the acceptance of "inferior professional service for the poor." Adelaide Nutting and Lavinia Dock, *A History of Nursing* (New York: G. P. Putnam's Sons, 1912), 3:25–26. See also Mary Gardner, *Public Health Nursing* (New York: Macmillan, 1916), 15–17.

In Canada, a similar system of district nursing was established by royal charter in 1897. There the Victorian Order of Nurses was founded as the National Memorial of the Diamond Jubilee of Queen Victoria. Based for all practical purposes along the same lines as the Jubilee Institute, the Canadian nurses even wore the same uniforms and insignia as the Queen's nurses. The Victorian Order's headquarters were established in Ottawa, with training centers in Montreal and Toronto. Like their English counterparts, these nurses were required to have training in both the hospital and the home. The first year, 14 nurses were admitted and 5 districts opened. By 1904, 35 branches and 90 nurses were working throughout the country. By the same time in the United States, there were 220 district nursing associations employing 537 nurses and 698 associations with 1,500 nurses in the British Isles. See Yssabella Waters, "The Rise, Progress, and Extent of Visiting Nurses in the United States," *Charities and the Commons* 16 (April 1906): 16–19; Hughes, "Rise of District Nursing"; and Margaret Allen, "Victorian Order of Nurses for Canada," *Charities and the Commons* 16 (April 1906): 19–21. See also Brainard, *Evolution*, 404–409.

24   See Carroll Smith-Rosenberg, *Religion and the Rise of the American City the New York City Mission Movement, 1812–1870* (Ithaca, N.Y.: Cornell University Press, 1971); and Nathan Huggins, *Protestants against Poverty: Boston's Charities, 1870–1900* (Westport, Conn.: Greenwood, 1971).

25   Boyer, *Urban Masses*, 143–161; Rosenberg, "Social Class and Medical Care in 19th Century America: The Rise and Fall of the Dispensary"; and Allen Davis, *Spearheads for Reform: The Social Settlements and the Progressive Movement, 1890–1914* (New York: Oxford University Press, 1967).

26   Brainard, *Evolution*, 195–202.

27   Ibid., 203–225. While these organizations were not the first to send out visiting nurses, they are often cited as the first, since providing skilled care for the sick poor was their sole purpose. See also C. E. M. Somerville, "District Nursing," in *Hospitals, Dispensaries and Nursing*, 539. For an early discussion of these activities, see Fulmer, "Visiting Nurse Work." For a more detailed account, see Brainard, *Evolution*, 194–261.

28   Brainard, *Evolution*, 203–214. See also Sarah Groves, "The Instructive District Nurse Association: 1885–1912" (MSN thesis, Boston University, 1970), 1–27. A staff member, a Miss Gordon, was apparently sent to London in 1887 to take the Metropolitan and National Nursing Association's three-month training course in district nursing. See Emile M. Monsel to Abbie Howes, December 12, 1885; and August 11, 1887, Instructive District Nurse Association (IDNA) Collection, Boston

University (hereafter cited as IDNA Collection), n34, box 1, folder 1; and Secretary's notebook for January 19, 1886–1887, IDNA Collection, box 2, folder 1.

29 Brainard, *Evolution*. The budget for the first year was $2,222. IDNA of Boston, *Annual Report* (1886).

30 Brainard, *Evolution*, 214–225; and Visiting Nurse Society (VNS) of Philadelphia, *Annual Report* (1887). By the end of March 1887, VNS had two nurses and three helpers who had made a total of 5,885 visits.

31 Brainard, *Evolution*, 218–219.

32 For an excellent discussion of Hampton and her influence on both district nursing and the profession in general, see Janet Wilson James, "Isabel Hampton and the Professionalization of Nursing in the 1890s," in *The Therapeutic Revolution: Essays in the Social History of American Medicine*, ed. Morris Vogel and Charles Rosenberg (Philadelphia: University of Pennsylvania Press, 1979), 201–244.

33 Welch was interested in creating a major institute of hygiene in Baltimore as early as 1884. He was active in public health in Baltimore and in the nation. He was involved in preventing the spread of a cholera epidemic in 1893, fought for sanitary reforms in Baltimore, and was elected to the State Board of Health in Maryland in 1898 and became its president in 1900. He played a major role in organizing the National Association for the Study and Prevention of Tuberculosis in 1904 and the National Committee for Mental Hygiene in 1908 and was instrumental in obtaining Rockefeller funding for the Johns Hopkins School of Hygiene and Public Health in 1916. See Elizabeth Fee, "Popsy's Baby," *Johns Hopkins Magazine* 34 (October 1983): 18–21; and Elizabeth Fee, "Competition for the First School of Hygiene and Public Health," *Bulletin of the History of Medicine* 57 (Fall 1983): 339–363.

34 James, "Hampton." Hampton describes her travels and subsequent views on district nursing in a paper she presented to the Annual Meeting of the Baltimore Charity Organization Society, 1891. The paper "District Nursing" appears in Isabel Hampton Robb, *Educational Standards for Nurses, with Other Addresses on Nursing Subjects* (Cleveland: E. C. Koeckert, 1907), 45–54.

35 James, "Hampton"; and Isabel Hampton, "Training Schools for Nurses," in *Proceedings of the National Conference of Charities and Correction at the Seventeenth Annual Session*, ed. Isabel C. Barrows (Boston: Geo. H. Ellis, 1890), 145–146.

36 James, "Hampton"; and Hampton, "District Nursing."

37 For Dock's account of these events, see Lavinia Dock, "Recollections of Miss Hampton at the Johns Hopkins," *AJN* 11 (October 1910): 18; and Nutting and Dock, *History of Nursing*, 3:125–127.

    In the winter of 1892, before the plans for the congress had fully crystallized, Ethel Gordon Fenwick, one of the leading British nurses and editor of the British journal *Nursing Record*, came to Chicago to arrange an exhibit of British nursing publications. Realizing the possibilities of the fair, she suggested a congress on nursing to the lady managers, who referred the matter to Billings. Helen Marshall, *Mary Adelaide Nutting: Pioneer of Modern Nursing* (Baltimore, Md.: Johns Hopkins University Press, 1972), 56–57.

38 Dock, "Recollections." Dock was one of the earliest visiting nurses in the country, having worked for a city mission in New York, among other things, before joining Hampton in Baltimore. For a discussion of her life and work, see "Authors in the Nursing Field: Lavinia Lloyd Dock," *Trained Nurse and Hospital Review* 76 (February 1926): 181; and Mary Roberts, "Lavinia Lloyd Dock—Nurse, Feminist, Internationalist," *AJN* 56 (February 1956): 176–179. On her return to London, Fenwick

stopped at Baltimore to visit Hopkins and to confer with Hampton and her associates, Dock and Nutting. Their discussions reportedly included nurses' associations, registration, standards for nursing schools, professional journals, and the way in which the Chicago World's Fair could be used to advance the cause of nursing in the United States and Canada. Unfortunately, Fenwick would not be able to attend the fair. Marshall, *Nutting*, 57.

39   As a result of her correspondence with Nightingale, Hampton convinced Nightingale to send a paper to the congress. Nightingale's paper "Sick Nursing and Health Nursing" was presented by Hampton as the keynote address and included a section on district nursing. Dock, "Recollections"; and Marshall, *Nutting*, 57. Hampton restated her views on district nursing in her paper "Educational Standards for Nurses," 33–34; Florence Nightingale, "Sick Nursing and Health Nursing," in *Nursing of the Sick, 1893*, ed. Isabel Hampton et al. (New York: McGraw-Hill, 1949), 444–463; Hughes, "Queen Victoria's Jubilee Institute," 531–539; Somerville, "District Nursing," in *Hospitals, Dispensaries and Nursing*, 539–547; and Mrs. Dacre Craven née Florence Lee, "On District Nursing," 547–554. All are included in Billings and Hurd, *Hospitals, Dispensaries and Nursing*.

40   The discussion that followed the papers on district nursing can be found on 554–556 of *Hospitals, Dispensaries and Nursing*.

41   Wald was greatly influenced by Craven and Nightingale's writings. Craven's work served as an important source for many earlier articles on nursing. Lagemann, *Generation of Women*, 68, 72. Lagemann also describes Wald's decision made in March 1893 to move to the Lower East Side and her first year there: see Lagemann, *Generation of Women*, 71–78. See also R. L. Duffus, *Lillian Wald: Neighbor and Crusader* (New York: Macmillan, 1939), 27–40. The congress was, no doubt, where Wald first met Dock and Hampton but not Nutting, who had remained in Baltimore having been left in charge while the others attended the congress. We know Wald attended because her comments are quoted in one of the discussions: see Billings and Hurd, *Hospitals, Dispensaries and Nursing*, 524. There were a few other less well-known nursing settlements organized during this period. See Brainard, *Evolution*, 250–261, and the series of articles on settlements in *Charities and the Commons* 16 (April 1906): 45–51.

42   James, "Hampton."

43   In 1912, the Cleveland ladies bequeathed the newly founded National Organization for Public Health Nursing (NOPHN) their insignia and their journal, the *Visiting Nurse Quarterly* (*VNQ*). But their greatest gift was Bolton, whose financial support made possible and whose opinions shaped much of the organization's activities. These events are discussed in chapters 4 and 5.

44   James, "Hampton"; and Roberts, "Lavinia." Dock visited Wald and Brewster while they were still living on Jefferson Street; see Duffus, *Wald*, 39; and Lagemann, *Generation of Women*, 79. While Hopkins's nursing programs did not include special training in this field for many years, pupils were encouraged to work with the staff of an established visiting nurse association (VNA) after graduation to gain some practical knowledge of the work before embarking upon it. Many chose the IDNA of Boston for this undertaking. See Board of Directors' meeting, April 19, 1895; and the IDNA of Boston, *Annual Report* (1895).

45   Evelyn Pope, the nurse who founded the Instructive VNA of Baltimore in 1896, was a Hopkins graduate and a classmate of Nutting's. Brainard, *Evolution*, 237. Ellen La Motte was director of the Tuberculosis Program at the Baltimore Health Department

and later the author of several books, including *Tuberculosis Nurse, Backwash of War, Peking Post, Civilization*, and *The Opium Monopoly and the Ethics of Opium. John Hopkins Nursing Alumni Magazine (JHNAM)* 25 (May 1926): 85. See also "Pioneers in Public Health: Ellen La Motte," *Trained Nurse and Hospital Review* (September 1928): 310. Fox worked at the Chicago VNS and then became director first of the Dayton, Ohio, and later of the Washington, DC, VNS. For twelve years she was director of the American Red Cross Public Health Nursing Service, leaving in 1930 to become executive director of the VNA in New Haven, Connecticut, and a member of the faculty of the Yale School of Nursing. From 1921 to 1926, she was president of the NOPHN. *JHNAM* 29 (May 1930): 64–66. Stevens guided the development of the Maternity Center Association in New York and in 1922 became general director of the NOPHN. M. Louise Fitzpatrick, *The National Organization for Public Health Nursing, 1912–1952: Development of a Practice Field* (New York: National League for Nursing, 1975), 93; and *JHNAM* 20 (November 1921): 265. Carr was Nutting's assistant at Hopkins and was later, for six years, director of the Instructive VNA of Baltimore. Later in her career, she became editor of the *Public Health Nurse (PHN)*, associate director of the NOPHN, and head of the Educational Department of the Instructive District Nursing Association (IDNA) of Boston. Blanche Pfefferkorn, "Ada Carr, 1893: A Remembrance," *JHNAM* 54 (October 1955): 152–153; and *JHNAM* 29 (November 1930): 212–215. Olmstead worked with Lent at the IDNA of Baltimore and then became state supervisor and director of the Public Health Nursing with the University of Wisconsin, a Red Cross nurse stationed in Europe during the war, and secretary for the NOPHN opening their Chicago office in 1918. Later she became assistant chief of the Department of Nursing and director of Public Health Nursing for the League of Red Cross Societies in Geneva. *JHNAM* 15 (May 1926): 87; and *JHNAM* 17 (November 1918): 228. Alta Dines worked with the maternity center and Henry Street Settlement, was director of the course in public health nursing at Western Reserve University, and later became director of Nursing Services with the Association for Improving the Condition of the Poor in New York. *PHN* 20 (April 1928): 198. Patterson was director of NOPHN and then became director of the Community Health Association (CHA) of Boston after Beard resigned. *JHNAM* 25 (May 1926): 86; and "Biographies of Candidates," *PHN* 18 (April 1926): 196. Waters joined Wald at the Henry Street Settlement and became the first statistician of the field. Her earliest publication was the survey *Visiting Nursing in the United States* (New York: Chanties, 1909). Finally, Lent was for thirteen years superintendent of the Instructive VNA of Baltimore and then joined the staff of NOPHN. She was sent to reorganize public health nursing in Los Angeles and subsequently to the U.S. Public Health Service, where she helped organize the "Sanitary Zones" surrounding the army camps in this country. After the war, she continued her work with NOPHN until she left nursing in 1922 to open an antique store. "Mary E. Lent: A Pioneer in Public Health Nursing," *JHNAM* 46 (April 1947): 60–62.

46 Marshall, *Nutting*, 63, 122, 79, 96, 154, 168–169; and Teresa Christy, *Cornerstone for Nursing Education: A History of the Division of Nursing Education of Teachers College Columbia University, 1899–1947* (New York: Teachers College Press, 1969), 34–41. In 1909, through an endowment given by Mrs. Helen Hurtley Jenkins, no doubt as a result of Wald s influence, the program of study was expanded, creating the Department of Nursing and Health. The curriculum included hygiene and sanitation, health problems, and social psychology. Brainard, *Evolution*, 316–318. See also Adelaide Nutting, "Nursing and Health," *VNQ* 2 (April 1910): 10.

47 By 1905, there were 171 associations hiring 445 visiting nurses, and by 1921, there were over eleven thousand public health nurses. Brainard, *Evolution*, 226, 428–432; and Fulmer, "Visiting Nurse Work," 413.

48 Wald relates some of her earlier experiences with doctors in Wald, *House on Henry Street*, 30–38. See also VNS of Philadelphia, *Annual Report* (1901); and Gardner, *Public Health Nursing*, 43–46.

49 For an excellent discussion of the changing nature of the voluntary hospital, see Rosner, *Once Charitable Enterprise*; and Vogel, *Modern Hospital*. For a discussion of the visiting nurse's role in reducing hospital costs, see Fulmer, "Visiting Nurse Work"; and "The Hospital Deficit," *Trained Nurse and Hospital Review* 32 (February 1904): 115. See, for example, Haven Emerson to Lillian Wald, December 9, 1905, Wald Collection, New York Public Library (hereafter cited as Wald Collection), roll 8. In 1887, the Philadelphia Board of Managers sent a circular to local physicians and the president of Public Charities explaining how the visiting nurse could provide comfort to patients who could not be admitted to Philadelphia General Hospital and also enable some who were already in the hospital to go home. The end result, they argued, would be less expensive for the city. Board of Managers Meeting, VNS of Philadelphia, October 21, 1887.

50 Shawe, *Notes for Visiting Nurses*, 10–18; Jacques, *District Nursing*, 32–42; Fulmer, "Visiting Nurse Work"; LaMotte, *The Tuberculosis Nurse: Her Function and Her Qualifications* (New York: G. P. Putnam's Sons, 1915), 11–19; and District Nurse Association (DNA) of Providence, *Annual Report* (1911), 28. With the exception of the IDNA of Boston, it is impossible to determine where visiting nurses trained or their previous work experience. This information is included in IDNA, *Annual Report* (1905), 6–7; and (1906), 6–9. Most of the staff were graduates of large general hospitals and one or more specialty hospitals. Most had previous hospital experience as head nurses or had done private duty. While several were from Canada, New York, Chicago, and Rhode Island, more than half trained in Boston.

51 "Visiting Nurse—a Ministry of All the Talents," *VNQ* 3 (April 1911): 27–31; Shawe, *Notes for Visiting Nurses*, 10–16, 26–27; and May Anna Tomlinson, "Compensation in Visiting Nursing," *PHNQ* 6 (January 1914): 77–78.

52 Mary Gardner in DNA of Providence, *Annual Report* (1911), 29.

53 Many had a three-month probation period to try to prevent so much turnover. For example, in 1906, there were only five (out of sixteen) nurses in the Philadelphia staff that had been there for more than two years. That same year, twelve nurses had resigned: one to marry, two because of "ill health," some to take up more lucrative positions, and others to help their families. "Report of the Head Nurse," VNS of Philadelphia, *Annual Report* (1906). This was not a new or uncommon problem. See, for example, Board of Managers Meeting for June 1, 1894; June 7, 1895; and April 2, 1897. Harriet Fulmer tried to introduce the topic of nurses' hesitancy to enter the field at the Nurses' Associated Alumnae of United States Meeting, but apparently the participants were not the least interested in discussing it. See Harriet Fulmer, "The Theory and Practice of Visiting Nursing, and the Attitude of the Profession towards It," *AJN* 6 (July 1906): 821–823; Wald, *House on Henry Street*, 42–43; and "Supervisor's Report," *VNQ* 1 (January 1909): 19.

54 Wald, *House on Henry Street*, 28.

55 Shawe, *Notes for Visiting Nurses*, 28–29.

56 Ibid.; Lillian Wald, "The Treatment of Families in Which There Is Sickness," *AJN* 4 (December 1904): 427–431.

57 Wald, *House on Henry Street*, 42; and Wald, "Treatment of Families." See, for example, IDNA of Boston, *Annual Report* (1902), 13; (1903), 15; and (1904), 17.

58 See the VNS of Philadelphia, "Report" for 1892.

59 Wald, "Treatment of Families," 431.

60 VNS, "Report."

61 Shawe, *Notes for Visiting Nurses*, 28–29.

62 This issue was chosen as the first topic for discussion at what has been described as "the first really representative gathering of visiting nurses" held at the invitation of the National Conference of Charities and Correction in June 1904. The question was "Should the educational and instructive features of visiting nursing be given such importance as to make skilled nursing only a secondary consideration?" The participants, having "thoroughly ventilated the question," finally concluded that "the two must go hand in hand, but that as valuable and essential as education and instruction are, they cannot take this place of nursing care." There had apparently been some public criticism of district nursing methods that led to this discussion. Ada Carr, "Visiting Nurses at the National Conference of Charities and Correction," *JHNAM* 3 (July 1904): 136–140. Wald certainly agreed, seeing instruction as an incidental consideration. Wald, *House on Henry Street*, 27. The subsequent evolution of this issue is discussed in chapters 3 and 5.

63 IDNA of Boston, *Annual Report* (1902), 13; (1903), 15; and (1905), 17. For comparison, see VNS of Philadelphia, *Annual Report* (1899), 12; (1904), 9; and (1905), 11; and DNA of Providence, *Annual Report* (1906), 21. For a list of specific diseases treated, see INDA of Boston, *Annual Report* (1909), 15.

64 Philadelphia had a higher proportion of German immigrants than Boston. Germans were seen in a much more positive light by the visiting nursing associations (VNAs), who described them as thrifty or good. See, for example, DNA of Providence, *Annual Report* (1910), 26; Nurses' Report, VNA of Dayton, Ohio (1902); or Boston University Nursing Archives (hereafter cited as Nursing Archive), n84, box 2, folder 11. While in Philadelphia and Boston, "Americans" constituted about 20 percent of the nurse's caseload; this group represented 44 percent of patients treated in Providence. It was not uncommon for these lists of nationalities to include the category "colored" as a separate listing from "American" and to include the categories "Jews" or "Jewish." IDNA of Boston, *Annual Report* (1909), 14–15; VNS of Philadelphia, *Annual Report* (1899), 7; (1904), 11; (1905), 12; and DNA of Providence, *Annual Report* (1905), 21; and Harriet Leet, "The Problem of Many Tongues," *VNQ* 2 (July 1910): 30–39; "The New District Nurse," *PHNQ* 5 (January 1913): 48–53; Helen Hempstead, "The Little Submerged Patient," *VNQ* 2 (July 1910): 41–45; and Harriet Mullony, "Less Familiar Friends from Central Europe," *PHNQ* 5 (July 1913): 99–114.

65 For nurses' views of the various nationalities, see Amy Potts, "Visiting Nursing in Philadelphia," *Trained Nurse and Hospital Review* 29 (August 1902): 85–88; Nurses' Report, VNA of Dayton (1902), Nursing Archive, n84, box 2, folder 11; "The Nurse's Story," DNA of Providence, *Annual Report* (1905), 14–15; "Report of the Superintendent," DNA of Providence, *Annual Report* (1910), 24–26; and "Editorial Comment," *VNQ* 1 (April 1909): 7–9; "Quarterly Report of Visiting Nurse Association," *VNQ* 1 (April 1909): 52–53, includes a survey conducted in sixty homes describing in some detail living conditions, diet, and so on. These views were not unique to nurses; see, for example, Joseph Mayper, "The Immigrant," *PHNQ* 5 (July 1913): 89–98.

66   Fulmer, "Visiting Nurse Work," 411–425; Beard, "Home Nursing," 44–47; Brainard, *Evolution*, 211; DNA of Providence, *Annual Report* (1908), 20; and Wald, *House on Henry Street*, 152–153.

67   Leet, "Problem of Many Tongues."

68   While one nurse in Cleveland claimed she cared for children of thirty-seven different nationalities, from the data available in several associations' annual reports, seventeen seems a more reasonable number.

        (See note 57.) Wald, "Treatment of Families," 430. One early editorial compared the visiting nurse's task to the game of croquet in *Alice in Wonderland*, suggesting that "the whole thing was rather alive" and that one had to regulate one's play accordingly: "Groups of different nationalities succeed each other in the same localities with a certain definite regularity—they seep and flow over various parts of the city as if obeying some tidal flow, the origin of which is no doubt connected with opportunities for their own material betterment." "Editorial Comment," *VNQ* 2 (April 1909): 7–9.

69   Wald, *House on Henry Street*, 42; and Fulmer, "Visiting Nurse Work."

70   Fulmer, "Visiting Nurse Work," 413–414.

71   Most of what we know of these early visiting nurses' work is based on books or annual reports. While some annual reports from Boston contained what were called "specimen pages, from weekly records of the nurses, filed at the office," these tended to be more complete than the few remaining unpublished reports written by staff. No matter what the source, the nurses' interventions seem consistent. The major concern of most nurses remained air, sunshine, windows, washing, spitting, and wounds; good air was seen as an especially important part of good health, evoking all sorts of techniques for converting believers. One of the best was a catechism entitled "The Air," which appeared in the *VNQ* 2 (January 1910): 31–32.

"The Air"

1.   Is fresh air good for me? I cannot live without it.
2.   Is air ever bad? Yes, it gets poisonous.
3.   What makes it poisonous? Every time anyone breathes, he throws poisons into the air.
4.   What are these poisons like? Some are poisonous gases; some like tiny poison seeds.
5.   Will they hurt me? They will kill one in time.
6.   How can I avoid these poisons? By always keeping in fresh air.

For "specimen pages," see IDNA of Boston, *Annual Report* (1902), 28–29; (1903), 30–31; and (1900), 14–15. For data on numbers of cases and visits, see note 5. For more details about the nurses' work, see, for example, Nurses' Notes IDNA of Boston; "Work at Large," May 21, 1906; Mary Brown's write-up of her day's work at Henry Street, titled "Henry Street Visiting Nurse Service," November 1918, Boston University Archives, n9, box 6, folder 5; Somerville, "District Nursing," in *Hospitals, Dispensaries and Nursing*, 541; or Shawe, *Notes for Visiting Nurses*, 80–100. Shawe also lists the contents of the visiting nurse's bag and discusses her "dress," 35–45. In general, this is a book that told the nurse entering the field everything she needed to know. See also "Nurse Stories" that regularly appeared in the *VNQ*—for example, *VNQ* 1 (January 1909): 24–33; or "Stories Told by Nurses," *VNQ* 3 (July 1911): 71–83.

72 Somerville, "District Nursing." These nurses were paid $50–$60 per month, plus $5 for carfare. IDNA of Boston, *Annual Report* (1907), 11; and Fulmer, "Visiting Nurse Work," 413.

73 The canary is mentioned in the IDNA of Boston, *Annual Report* (1903), 20. The monkey story is part of an amusing leather-bound, handwritten and illustrated book by Miss R. King, for Mary Minot, one of the lady managers. Since there is no note of Miss King in the twentieth-century annual reports, she apparently wrote this book prior to that time. In the monkey story, she describes an "apparition like a feather-bed tied in the middle" who called for the nurse because her son was sick. Finding that he had measles—a "catching disease"—she quickly exposed the other children, declaring "me no care, all de chillen sick one time, one trouble." While its spread through the children was acceptable, when it came to the monkey, the source of the family's income, this was "too much trouble, too muchy sick." In the kitchen, the nurse found the monkey "crouched up in one corner of his box, with his head buried in his hands, his eyes running water." Covering his cage with a skirt, the nurse prescribed plenty of milk and water for the monkey. Visiting daily, she saved the monkey and won over the family. The book is in the IDNA Collection, n34, box 2.

74 Fulmer, "Visiting Nurse Work," 424; and Somerville, "District Nursing," in *Hospitals, Dispensaries and Nursing*, 539.

Chapter 2 — Trained Nurses for the Sick Poor

1 Mrs. J. H. Lowman, "Report on Co-operation," *VNQ* 4 (January 1912): 71–72. The association—which at that time had a staff of only five nurses—had thirty board members.

2 Ibid. Attending to both the patient and the room were of nearly equal importance to the early visiting nurses and followed carefully the teachings of Nightingale. See chapter 1. For instruction in both, see the popular text followed by most nurses, Craven, *Guide to District Nurses*. See also Florence Nightingale, *Notes on Nursing: What It Is, and What It Is Not* (London: Harrison, 1859). For a discussion of these ideas, see Charles Rosenberg, "Florence Nightingale on Contagion: The Hospital as Moral Universe," in *Healing and History: Essays for George Rosen*, ed. Charles Rosenberg (New York: Science History Publications, 1979), 116–136.

3 Lowman, "Report on Co-operation," 72.

4 Mary Gardner, "Twenty-Five Years Ago," *PHN* 29 (January 1937): 141–144.

5 Since a certain degree of expansion was required to create the issues, this chapter must by definition focus on the larger association. In 1909, this would include any association employing more than ten nurses: Providence, Rhode Island (seventeen); Brooklyn, New York (thirteen); Washington, DC (twelve); Baltimore, Maryland (fifteen); Boston (twenty-four); Henry Street, New York (fifty); Cleveland, Ohio (twenty-nine); and Philadelphia (nineteen). Waters, *Visiting Nursing*, 315–364.

6 Some of the agencies existing in 1901 are described in Fulmer, "Visiting Nurse Work." For the number of nurses employed by each association and the number of new associations each year, see Waters, *Visiting Nursing*, 315–365. A general description of the turn-of-the-century visiting nurse association (VNA) can be found in Gardner, "Twenty-Five Years Ago."

7 Katherine Tucker, "The Relationship between the Board and Its Professional Staff," *PHN* 19 (June 1927): 295.

8 It was not always easy to sustain a high level of enthusiasm and attendance. In most cities, as Brainard noted, "every man and woman of prominence is usually overburdened with civic and social duties." Accordingly, she suggested that if boards were large—with up to forty members—then at least twenty-five members be counted on to attend the meetings. Annie Brainard, "The Administrative Side of Visiting Nursing," *PHNQ* 7 (January 1915): 57–96.

9 Ibid., 66–67. For a similar discussion related to the selection of a board, see Gardner, *Public Health Nursing*, 100–112. For a complete listing of board members, see the annual reports of the association. But, for example, the Philadelphia board included such women as Mrs. Henry Lea, Mrs. William Furness Jenks, and the granddaughters of Lucretia Mott. Cordner, Mrs. William Sedgwick, and Mrs. Codman were among the early members of the Boston board.

10 See Brainard, *Evolution*, 203–249; and C. E. M. Somerville, "District Nursing," in *Nursing of the Sick*, 119–127. This paper discusses the early management of Boston's Instructive District Nursing Association (IDNA). The Providence District Nursing Association (DNA), which had a smaller number of nurses and managers, was organized in a similar fashion. The managers who worked directly with the nurses were often members of the committee on supervision of nurses or what was often simply called the "nurses' committee." See, for example, Mary Gardner, "A Successful Plan of Organization," *PHNQ* 5 (January 1913): 20–21. See also "Historical Notes from the Secretaries Minutes of the Nurse Committee's Meetings," DNA of Providence; Mary Aldis, "The Relationship of Directors and Nurses," *PHNQ* 5 (July 1913): 115–117; and Minutes of the Managers Meeting, Visiting Nurse Society (VNS) of Philadelphia, October 29, 1886; and May 1888.

11 Beard, "Home Nursing," 44–51.

12 This influence or corrective experience was frequently mentioned in the writings of lady managers. See, for example, One of the Older Women, "A Decade of Change," *PHNQ* 5 (January 1913): 68; and by One of Them [Mrs. John Lowman], "Concerning a Few of the Duties and Privileges of Trustees," *VNQ* 4 (April 1912): 25.

13 Beard, "Home Nursing," 45.

14 Tucker, "Relationship Between." May Aldis, president of the Chicago VNA, describes each nurse as feeling like she could go to her director sure of a friend. She also talks about the work of the "saving committee" in the same article, which kept back a small portion of the nurse's check each month. This could only be withdrawn with the approval of the committee. Although, she admitted, this might seem like mothering, the nurses were always grateful in the end. See Aldis, "Directors and Nurses," 117. John Lowman discusses the unlikely proposition of trying to bring these two groups together on a more equal basis by appointing staff members to the board as "the comingling of diverse elements, the materially free but spiritually bound, with the materially bound and spiritually free." In John Lowman, "Boards of Directors," *PHNQ* 5 (July 1913): 52.

15 Beard, "Home Nursing," 45.

16 Minutes of the Managers Meeting, VNS of Philadelphia, January 26, 1887. Linda Richards, who was the head nurse in Philadelphia for six months in 1891, was an exception to the typical head nurse–board member relationship. Miss Richards was seen as occupying a place unambiguously above the other nurses. Although it was realized her stay would be brief, in November 1891, the board elected her a member. Minutes of the Managers Meeting, VNS of Philadelphia, February 1891. Miss Richards briefly comments on her time in Philadelphia in her reminiscences,

recalling that at the time, it was a branch of work new to her "but which has been productive of much good, and which has called into service many of our noblest women who have found it the most attractive and interesting of all work yet entered upon by nurses." Linda Richards, *Reminiscences of Linda Richards: America's First Trained Nurse* (Boston: M. Barrow, 1929), 102.

17   Minutes of the Managers Meeting, VNS of Philadelphia, January 1888. Her salary was $900 per year.

18   Ibid., May 1888.

19   "Rules for the Nurses," VNS of Philadelphia, May 1888.

20   Minutes of the Managers Meeting, VNS of Philadelphia, June 1888.

21   VNS of Philadelphia, *Annual Report* (1888). The only explanation given in the annual report is that the ladies wished to do as in England and have the nurses live in the house. But in the minutes, it states that the desire to take over the whole house had resulted when "early in the summer it became apparent that in permitting the rooms connected with this office to be let to undergraduate doctors while young girls are employed as nurses could be a mistake." Minutes of the Managers Meeting, VNS of Philadelphia, Summer 1888.

22   Minutes of the Managers Meeting, VNS of Philadelphia, October 1888.

23   Ibid.

24   Ibid., October 1889.

25   "Rules for the Nurses," VNS of Philadelphia, July 1890.

26   Minutes of the Managers Meeting, VNS of Philadelphia, May 27, 1887; July 2, 1887; December 1, 1893; and April 7, 1916. One nurse was dismissed as unfit for the work despite her kindness of heart and willingness, another because she did work other than nursing for the patients.

27   Ibid., January 25, 1893; and February 1, 1895.

28   Gardner, "Plan of Organization," 20–28; Mary Gardner, "Our Executive Officers," *PHNQ* 5 (July 1913): 61–68; and Gardner, *Public Health Nursing*, 100–112.

29   Gardner, "Twenty-Five Years Ago," 141.

30   Mary Gardner, *Katharine Kent* (New York: Macmillan, 1946), 62.

31   Brainard, *Evolution*, 212.

32   Miss Beer's report, November 28, 1900, IDNA of Boston, Nursing Archives, n34, box 2, folder 3.

33   Brainard, *Evolution*, 212.

34   IDNA of Boston, *Annual Report* (1912), 24.

35   This is how the Philadelphia managers described their new superintendent. VNS of Philadelphia, *Annual Report* (1915), 5.

36   IDNA of Boston, *Annual Report* (1912), 16.

37   One of the Older Women, "Decade of Change," 67.

38   Ibid., 68.

39   Beard was a graduate of New York Hospital School of Nursing in 1903. Her career will be discussed in detail later. "Mary Beard Dies: Leader of Nurses," *New York Times*, December 5, 1946, 29. Gardner came from a prominent Providence family, was a graduate of Newport Hospital, and became superintendent of the DNA of Providence in 1905. Brainard, *Evolution*, 242. In Gardner, "Plan of Organization," 20–28, Gardner describes the organization she created in Providence. She discusses her early experiences as a superintendent in "Twenty-Five Years Ago," 141–144. Finally, in Gardner, "Our Executive Officers," 61–68, she discusses the duties of a superintendent. Foley was a 1901 graduate of Smith College, a graduate of the

Hartford Hospital Training School, and hired by the VNA of Chicago to reorganize that association in 1911. "Smith College Honors Miss Foley," *Trained Nurse and Hospital Review* 81 (July 1928): 199; and E. P. Crandall, "Memorandum in re Circumstances Leading to the Organization of National Organization for Public Health Nursing," Gardner Papers, Schlesinger Library, Radcliffe College (hereafter cited as Gardner Papers), folder 45.

40 Fox was a graduate of the University of Wisconsin and the Johns Hopkins School of Nursing. Her first experience in visiting nursing was at the VNA of Chicago with Foley. In 1913, she was appointed the superintendent of the VNA of Dayton, Ohio, which was in the midst of a reorganization that ultimately resulted in the combining of the VNA staff with the Tuberculosis Society and the health department nurses into a single staff. This process is described in the VNA of Dayton, *Annual Reports* (1913 and 1914), Boston University Library, n84, box 2, folder 20, 21, 22. See also Elizabeth Holt, "Reorganization of Public Health Nursing in Dayton, Ohio," *PHN* 17 (September 1925): 520–522. Fox resigned in February 1915: "The call came from Washington to come and help reorganize the visiting nurse work there: she had been so successful in reorganizing our own association that we realized what it would mean to the work and standards, to have her accept the offer. Chicago came to our assistance again as she had so loyally in the past and sent us our new superintendent, Miss Elizabeth Holt." "Report of the Annual Meeting" for 1915, Dayton VNA, Boston University, n84, box 2, folder 23, p. 3. Fox's career is described in the *JHNAM* 29 (May 1930): 64–66. Lent was a graduate of the class of 1895 at Hopkins, and after being on the staff for several years, she became superintendent of the Instructive VNA of Baltimore in 1903. In July 1916, she went to Los Angeles to survey and reorganize the work of the public health nurse. At the time, she was the executive director of the National Organization for Public Health Nursing (NOPHN) and was "loaned" to the city for six months. "Mary E. Lent," 61. Tucker was a graduate of Vassar and did her nurses training at Newton Hospital. She began her nursing career as a tuberculosis worker at the university hospital and in 1912 became the head worker at the New York Dispensary. Between 1913 and 1916, she was director of the Social Service Department of the Mental Hygiene Committee of the New York State Charities Association and in 1916 became general director of the VNS of Philadelphia.

41 Ibid. The above footnote gives some indications of the interrelatedness of these women's careers. See also Gardner, "Twenty-Five Years Ago." Once the NOPHN had been formed, its encounters became even more numerous. For example, the reorganization in Dayton was done with consultation with Crandall, Matilda Johnson, Gardner, and Foley. By that time, Crandall was the executive secretary of the NOPHN; Johnson was a member of the NOPHN's first board; Gardner was secretary of the committee appointed to consider formation of the NOPHN, a member of the first board, and its president from 1913 to 1916; and Foley was chair of the committee to organize the NOPHN, its first vice president, and later its president. VNA of Dayton, *Annual Report* (1915), Boston University, n84, box 2, folder 22. See also Elizabeth Fox, "Methods of Establishing a Visiting Nurse Association," *PHNQ* 7 (January 1915): 82.

42 It was Crandall, who at the time was teaching at Teachers College, who suggested the Boston board consider first LaMotte and later Beard as potential superintendents. LaMotte was a member of the first board of the NOPHN, and Beard was a member of the committee appointed to consider the formation of the NOPHN, a

member of the first board of the NOPHN, and president, 1916–1919. Lent was the first treasurer of the NOPHN and its associate director, 1916–1921. Elizabeth Fox "The Past Challenges the Future," *PHN* 29 (May 1937): 279. It is interesting to note, but not very surprising, that many of the early leaders in this field were Hopkins graduates. As James has demonstrated, Hopkins's widespread reputation made it possible to attract a very different kind of woman to nursing, one with a strong education background and prominent social position. The early Hopkins students came from middle- to upper-middle-class families, and few were dependent upon their salaries for a livelihood. In addition, there was ample encouragement for Hopkins students to become visiting nurses. Isabel Hampton, the first superintendent at Hopkins, recognized, according to James, "the potentialities of a new kind of work which would both fulfill woman's mission of social uplift and enhance the status of nurses." James, "Isabel Hampton and the Professionalization of Nursing in the 1890s," 213–214, 226–227. Other members of this generation of visiting nurse leaders who graduated from Hopkins include Katharine Olmstead, LaMotte, Carr, Waters, Florence Patterson, and Stevens.

43 Rosenberg, "Inward Vision and Outward Glance," 346–391; Rosner, *Once Charitable Enterprise*; and Vogel, *Modern Hospital*.

44 In 1870, for example, operating expenses at Massachusetts General Hospital were $62,000; by 1910, they had gone to $350,300. The average cost per patient/day increased from $1.43 to $3.59 during the same period. Morris Vogel, "The Transformation of the American Hospital, 1850–1920," in *Health Care in America: Essays in Social History*, ed. Susan Reverby and David Rosner (Philadelphia: Temple University Press, 1979), 112. At Brooklyn Hospital, the average cost per day in 1915 was $2.78. Turn-of-the-century Brooklyn Hospital had debts ranging from $27,000 to $75,000. Rosner, "Business at the Bedside," 120–121. In contrast, the cost per visit for a visiting nurse in 1911 was $0.50, and while many VNAs had deficits regularly, they were, by comparison, small—$3,000 to $5,000. Their expenses were also much smaller, averaging $40,000 by 1910. See footnotes 81–85, chapter 2.

45 Dr. Hugh Cabot to Miss Elizabeth Cordner, February 25, 1908, IDNA Collection, n34, box 1, folder 2, pp. 1–2.

46 Ibid., 3–5.

47 IDNA of Boston, *Annual Report* (1908 and 1911). Unfortunately, as their expenses increased, their income decreased. In 1911, the board reported that during the past five years their expenses had increased by $22,000, while their income had decreased by $5,000. That year the association reported a deficit of $5,784. IDNA of Boston, *Annual Report* (1911), 19.

48 At the time, IDNA had forty-three staff nurses: ten maternity nurses, eleven Boston dispensary nurses, one nursery nurse, one industrial nurse, thirteen nurses working with private doctors, six Metropolitan Life Insurance Company (MLI) nurses, and one contagion nurse. On February 15, 1911, the board held a conference to discuss these problems and plan for the future. The conclusions were published in a "descriptive pamphlet." "Conference on District Nursing Problems, 2/16/11," IDNA Collection, n34, box 2, folder 3; IDNA of Boston, *Annual Reports* (Boston, 1912), 22; and "An Address," 11/11/11, IDNA Collection, n34, box 2, folder 3, p. 6.

49 Michael Davis to Mrs. E. A. Codman, April 27, 1911, IDNA Collection, n34, box 1, folder 3.

50 Ibid.

51 As a result of their conference, they decided that some type of "organic union" of the various unrelated groups of nurses should be created. First, they would combine the different specialized groups of IDNA nurses, and by summer, they hoped to unify the IDNA and the Baby Hygiene Association, an outcome that in fact required another ten years. "Conference on District Nursing," IDNA Collection; and IDNA of Boston, *Annual Report* (1911), 9.

52 Ella Crandall to Mrs. E. A. Codman, November 9, 1911, IDNA Collection, n34, box 1, folder 3.

53 Ida Cannon to Mrs. E. A. Codman, February 15, 1911; Edna Foley to Mrs. E. A. Codman, June 28, 1911; Ella Crandall to Mrs. E. A. Codman, August 25, 1911; and Ellen LaMotte to Mrs. E. A. Codman, September 26, 1911; and October 3, 1911, IDNA Collection, box 1, folder 3.

54 Elizabeth Ring Elliot to Mrs. E. A. Codman, n.d. (probably summer 1911); Ella Crandall to Mrs. Codman, August 31, 1911; Mary Goodville to Mrs. Codman and Gertrude Peabody to Mrs. Codman, n.d.; and Mary Lent to Mrs. Codman, September 14, 1911, IDNA Collection, box 1, folder 3.

55 Ella Crandall to Mrs. Codman, November 9, 1911. The board did not immediately write Beard but instead wrote Crandall a second letter requesting more information about Beard. Crandall to Mrs. Codman, November 21, 1911, IDNA Collection, n34, box 1, folder 3.

56 Ibid.

57 Ella Crandall to Mrs. Codman, November 9, 1911.

58 John Lewis to Mrs. Codman, March 24, 1911. Irene Sutliffe, who had been superintendent when Beard was a student at New York Hospital, wrote the board that Beard had a credible record and was a well-bred, intelligent woman with "a thoroughly social point of view." She did not think she had "great ability" but would do well as a head worker in a nursing association, "as she is in many ways fitted for that kind of work." Irene Sutliffe to Mrs. Codman, December 21, 1911, IDNA Collection, n34, box 1, folder 3. One cannot help but wonder if the underlying message was that she was fitted for visiting nursing but not so capable in other types of nursing.

59 IDNA of Boston, *Annual Report* (1912), 16, 23.

60 Mary Beard, "Report of the Work during June, 1912," IDNA of Boston.

61 IDNA of Boston, *Annual Report* (1912), 14–24.

62 IDNA of Boston, *Annual Report* (1914), 8.

63 IDNA of Boston, *Annual Report* (1913), 18, 24.

64 Ibid.

65 IDNA of Boston, *Annual Report* (1912), 25–27.

66 IDNA of Boston, *Annual Report* (1913), 22.

67 IDNA of Boston, *Annual Report* (1914), 10.

68 IDNA of Boston, *Annual Report* (1915), 16.

69 IDNA of Boston, *Annual Report* (1913), 19.

70 Ibid., 20–21.

71 Ibid., 20; Editorial, "The Atlantic City Meeting," *PHNQ* 5 (July 1913): 5–12; Florence Patterson, "The First Annual Meeting of the National Organization for Public Health Nursing," *PHNQ* 5 (July 1913): 13–19.

72 Fitzpatrick discusses this controversy in *National Organization*, 34. Beard's views were first published that year. Mary Beard, "Generalization in Public Health Nursing," *PHNQ* 5 (October 1913): 42–47. This debate continued well into the 1920s

and was one of the issues addressed by the Goldmark Report and the East Harlem Nursing Project. East Harlem Nursing and Health Service, *A Comparative Study of Generalized and Specialized Health Services* (New York: East Harlem Nursing and Health Service, 1926); and Josephine Goldmark, *Nursing and Nursing Education in the United States* (New York: Macmillan, 1923).

73 IDNA of Boston, *Annual Report* (1913), 20.

74 Ibid., 23; (1914), 14; and (1915), 26.

75 See the Treasurer's Report, IDNA of Boston, *Annual Report* (1914, 1915, and 1916). During the same period, the number of patients whose care was paid by MLI increased from 20 percent to 28 percent of all patients visited, but the percent of the association's total expenses contributed by the company decreased from 22 percent to 19.6 percent. Donations increased only slightly from $19,491 in 1911 to $22,617 by 1915 but failed to increase in proportion to the budget. To summarize, while expenses increased by 43 percent, income from donations increased 16 percent, income from MLI increased 20 percent, and income from patient out-of-pocket fees increased threefold.

76 IDNA of Boston, *Annual Report* (1911 and 1915).

77 See the Treasurer's Report, IDNA of Boston, *Annual Report* (1911 and 1915). The $17,000 represents the increased cost for all nurses, while increased cost for staff nurses alone was $13,914.

78 IDNA of Boston, *Annual Report* (1912), 20.

79 See Treasurer's Report, IDNA of Boston, *Annual Reports* (1911–1915).

80 Supervisors Meeting, IDNA of Boston, November 23, 1917. Tucker describes the transformation in the relationship between the managers and the nurses as a second stage, which in theory and practice proved unsound but was a necessary step before "a partnership of equals" and free of patronage in either direction could be created. Tucker, "Relationship Between."

81 For example, IDNA's turn-of-the-century deficits were usually a few hundred dollars—or at the worst, in 1903, $1,325. See the annual reports for complete financial statements.

82 By One of Them, "Concerning a Few," 25.

83 DNA of Providence, *Annual Report* (1910), 19; Brainard, "Administrative Side," 73–81.

84 The Boston Association had a budget of $53,000 and Chicago a budget of $85,000 as early as 1912. Lee Frankel, "Visiting Nursing from a Business Organization's Standpoint," *PHNQ* 5 (July 1913): 25–45.

85 The Philadelphia association decided to appoint an advisory board of men in 1914 to help them primarily with financial questions. Minutes of the Managers Meeting, VNS of Philadelphia, November 6, 1914. But unfortunately, it was not soon enough, since according to the annual report of 1915, "insufficient funds due to various business changes which caused a loss of over $4,000 income during the first 6 months of the fiscal year" had an "appalling deficit." This section, "The Great Debt," went on to say that the association was eventually saved by a benefit performance of the Battle Cry of Peace, generous friends who came forward, and the managers who took "much pains to raise money." VNS of Philadelphia, *Annual Report* (1915), 4. The Providence association faced an uncertain financial outlook by 1915 when its surplus was almost exhausted, while its yearly income was not sufficient to meet expenses. Faced with having to curtail services, they decided to go to the city to seek money to support their services for children. They also decided to reduce

the size of the annual report as an economy measure. DNA of Providence, *Annual Report* (1915), 7. In Boston, the IDNA reported in 1911 that during the past five years, their expenses had increased by $22,500, while their income had decreased by $5,000. IDNA of Boston, *Annual Report* (1911), 19. By December 1913, the situation had become so serious that in one section of the town, 118 volunteers conducted a house-to-house campaign, raising $11,953 for the association. Although this method troubled some of their oldest and best friends, those involved saw it as simply explaining their work to individuals and asking for their support. IDNA of Boston, *Annual Report* (1913), 13.

86   One of the Older Women, "Decade of Change," 67.

87   Gardner's patient classification system can be found in the DNA of Providence, *Annual Report* (1914), 29.

88   DNA of Providence, *Annual Report* (1909), 20; and VNS of Philadelphia, *Annual Report* (1907), 5. Philadelphia began to accept pay patients in 1888. These patients contributed $150 that year. VNS of Philadelphia, *Annual Report* (1888). The ladies were pleased with the nurses' results among the working class, noting in the report of 1892 that "it is not easy to exaggerate the educating influence of the visit of a trained nurse in a house where a high standard of cleanliness has never been seen and where ideas are on the level little above those of savages." VNS of Philadelphia, *Annual Report* (1892).

89   See, for example, DNA of Providence, *Annual Report* (1913), 26. By 1914, paying patients contributed $2,623 of a $32,000 budget. DNA of Providence, *Annual Report* (1914), 29. In 1912, $2,988 of Boston's $33,323 budget (6 percent) came from paying patients, while $12,065 (14 percent) of Chicago's $85,824 budget came from patients. Frankel, "Visiting Nursing," 27. Boston was able to increase its income from patients to 10 percent of the budget by 1917. IDNA of Boston, *Annual Report* (1917), 23, 27.

90   DNA of Providence, *Annual Report* (1914), 29. According to the Philadelphia managers, this type of work, often called "hourly nursing," seemed a "natural extension of the work of the Visiting Nurse Society" and had been "successfully consummated" by similar organizations in other cities. VNS of Philadelphia, *Annual Report* (1916). See also Editorial, "The Hourly Nurse," *Charities and the Commons* 16, no. 1 (April 1906): 3.

91   The origins and expansion of the MLI's nursing programs are described in Ella Crandall, "Memoranda on Circumstances Leading to the Organization of the National Organization for Public Health Nursing," May 1921, Gardner Papers, folder 45; MLI, *The Welfare Work of Metropolitan Life Insurance Company for Its Industrial Policyholders: Report 1915* (New York: MLI, 1915), 3; Lee Frankel, *Visiting Nursing and Life Insurance: Statistical Summary of Results of Eight Years* (New York: MLI, September 1911), 4; Ella Crandall, "A New Extension of Visiting Nursing," *AJN* 10 (January 1909): 236–239; and Alma Haupt, "Nursing and Life Insurance," MLI Archives, New York, folder titled "Papers and Speeches, Haupt, Alma," p. 471.

92   Grace Allison, "Shall Attendants Be Trained and Registered?," *AJN* 12 (August 1912): 333; DNA of Providence, *Annual Report* (1913), 37; and the VNS of Philadelphia, *Annual Report* (1911), 2. Income from the MLI constituted 20 percent of the budget in 1913. IDNA of Boston, *Annual Report* (1913), 44, 47.

93   Frankel, "Visiting Nursing." The ladies were willing to work on their record systems and might admit their nurses could make more visits each day, but Frankel went too far when he insisted that a prerequisite to attracting paying patients was to separate their association from charitable activities. At one point, Frankel went

so far as to suggest that this "charitable problem" could be solved for his policy-holders by giving MLI exclusive use of certain nurses, to be known as MLI nurses, who would wear a distinctive badge and eventually have a separate supervisor. In addition, he did not want it to be known that these "MLI nurses" were really working for the VNA; not surprisingly, visiting nurses were dismayed at the suggestion. Minutes of the Manger's Meeting, VNS of Philadelphia, December 19, 1912. The outcome was a categorical rejection of Frankel's proposal by the boards, even when faced with the possibility of MLI creating its own nursing service. This issue will be discussed in greater detail as it relates to the efforts of visiting nurses to raise their professional status in chapter 4.

94 Frankel, "Visiting Nursing," 25–45.

95 DNA of Providence, *Annual Report* (1913), 28–29. The IDNA annual report refers to his speech as "an admirable address" that pointed out "several things which we shall look forward to in the future," but it only goes on to mention his suggestion that visiting nursing should be supported by large corporations. IDNA of Boston, *Annual Report* (1913), 17.

Chapter 3 — The Hope and Promise of Public Health

1 George Rosen, *Preventive Medicine in the United States: 1900–1975, Trends and Interpretations* (New York: Prodist, 1977), 14–19.

2 Ibid.

3 Ibid., 47, 18–19; Michael Davis, *Immigrant Health and the Community* (New York: Harper Brothers, 1921); John Blake, *Origins of Maternal and Child Health Programs* (New Haven, Conn.: Department of Public Health, Yale University School of Medicine, 1953); and William Schmidt, "Development of Health Services for Mothers and Children in the United States," *AJPH* 8 (March 1908): 464–467.

4 "Their Health Is Your Health," a fundraising booklet for Henry Street Nurses' Settlement, 1934.

5 For further discussion of this new role, see C.-E. A. Winslow, "The Untilled Field of Public Health," *Science* 51 (January 1920): 23–33; and C.-E. A. Winslow, "The New Profession of Public Health Nursing and Its Educational Needs," speech, 1917, Winslow Collection, Yale University Library, New Haven, Conn. (hereafter cited as Winslow Collection), folder 119:129.

6 Nutting, "Nursing and Health," 10.

7 In his chapter titled "The New Public Health," Winslow describes education in the conduct of the individual life as the "dominant motive" of this campaign. The new public health movement was, according to Winslow, the third distinctive phase in the development of public health. It was preceded by the period of empirical environmental sanitation, which extended from 1840 to 1890, and the period of scientific control of communicable disease, which dominated the field between 1890 and 1910. C.-E. A. Winslow, *The Evolution and Significance of the Modern Public Health Campaign* (New Haven, Conn.: Yale University Press, 1935), 49–65.

8 John Ferrell, "The Trends of Preventive Medicine in the United States," *Journal of the American Medical Association* (*JAMA*) 81 (September 1923): 1063–1069; Lee Frankel, "Science and Public Health," *AJPH* 5 (April 1915): 281–289; Haven Emerson, "Meeting the Demand for Community Health Work," *PHN* 16 (September 1924): 487; and Winslow, *Evolution and Significance*, 49–65.

9 William Field, "Civic Control of Public Health Nursing," *PHNQ* 6 (October 1914): 70–80. Ibid.

10 Ibid. See also Charles Chapin, "The Evolution of Preventive Medicine," *JAMA* 76 (January 1921): 215–222. For a discussion of the changes in emphasis, see Rosenkrantz, *Public Health and the State*; and Barbara Rosenkrantz, "Cart before Horse: Theory, Practice and Professional Image in American Public Health, 1870–1920," *Journal of the History of Medicine and Allied Sciences* 29 (January 1974): 55–73. The most often mentioned source for the theory and practice of the new public health was Hibbert Hill, *The New Public Health* (New York: Macmillan, 1916). This book is summarized in Alice Hamilton and Gertrude Seymour's series entitled "The New Public Health," which appeared in *Survey* 37 (November 1916): 165–169; 37 (January 1917): 456–459; and 38 (April 1917): 59–62.

11 Winslow, *Evolution and Significance*, 52–55; and Charles Eliot, "The Main Points of Attack in the Campaign for Public Health," *AJPH* 5 (July 1915): 619–625.

12 Mary Lent, "The True Functions of the Tuberculosis Nurse," *Transactions of the Sixth International Congress on Tuberculosis* (*TICTB*; 1908): 576.

13 Winslow, *Evolution and Significance*, 52. Thus knowledge could be communicated directly to "mothers who bring up the babies and the men who pay the rent in the tenements and work in the stores and factories." Ibid., 55. See also Emerson, "Meeting the Demand."

14 Nightingale, "Sick Nursing and Health Nursing," 24–42. Wald claimed that the idea of the modern "public health nurse found its inception in the mind of Nightingale." Wald Collection, box 32, *New York Times Magazine*, January 26, 1919, p. 10.

15 Nightingale, "Sick Nursing and Health Nursing." These were her last published works on nursing. Florence Nightingale, "Health Teaching in Towns and Villages: Rural Hygiene," in *Selected Writings of Florence Nightingale*, 377–396. See also W. J. Bishop, *A Bio-bibliography of Florence Nightingale* (London: Dawsons of Pall Mall, 1962), 14, 33–35, 132.

16 Nightingale, "Health Teaching."

17 George Rosen, *A History of Public Health* (New York: MD Publications, 1958), 376–378. For a brief history of health visitors in England, see Rosemary Hale, *The Principles and Practice of Health Visiting* (Oxford: Pergamon, 1966), 7–16; and Florence Greenwood, "The Evolution of the Health Visitor," *Journal of Royal Sanitary Institute* 34 (February 1913): 174–182.

18 During World War I, this distinction would be critical when health officers attempted to replace the public health nurse with a nonnurse health visitor. See, for example, E. V. Baumbaugh, "The Public Health Instructor: A New Type of Health Worker," *AJPH* 8 (August 1918): 662–664. This situation is discussed in more detail in chapter 4. See also Lillian Wald, "Educational Value and Social Significance of the Trained Nurse in the Tuberculosis Campaign," *TICTB* (1908): 637; and Charlotte Aikens, "The Educational Opportunity of the Visiting Nurse in the Prevention of Disease," in *Proceedings of the National Conference of Charities and Corrections at the Thirty-Third Annual Session*, ed. Alexander Johnson (n.p.: Press of Fred J. Heer, n.d.), 185–195. Physicians shared this view. See, for example, Emerson, "Meeting the Demand"; and Chapin, "Evolution of Preventive Medicine."

19 Winslow, "New Profession."

20 Lent, "True Functions." For example, one tuberculosis nurse describing her frustrations with physicians, decried those whose treatment of tuberculosis still depended "on cod liver oil and a change of climate: who never think to advise a patient how to care for his sputum or pay attention to the conditions of his home." Marie Phelon, "The Disinfection of Houses: What Is Not Done," *TICTB* (1908): 502.

21 Winslow, "Untilled Field." For an interesting discussion of these developments, see Barbara Melosh, *The Physician's Hand: Work, Culture and Conflict in American Nursing* (Philadelphia: Temple University Press, 1982), 113–157.

22 "An Ancient Occupation and a Modern Profession," *PHN* 11 (January 1919): 12.

The Health Department Nurse

Where the cooling breeze never seem to come,
   Where the summer heat is throbbing out its nurse,
Where the stench of human living marks the slum,
   There is where you'll find the Health Department Nurse.

Where the garbage-littered alleys ooze and smell,
   Where the old-faced children swarm the narrow street,
Where is found the human dump, a living hell,
   Where they're slaving on but half enough to eat

Where the summer death-rate claims its highest toll,
   Where every sixth or seventh baby dies,
Where slattern mothers count the mournful roll
   That is yearly called to fever, filth and flies.

Here—where public greed and ignorance play a part
   To the pulling of the politician's strings,
Does the Health Nurse find her work and break her heart
   With the aching of the gladness that she brings.

Here, in spotless white, amid disease and grime,
   Is she carrying the gospel of the clean
And a ray dawning health will mark the time,
   For they're hungry for the chance that they have seen.
To the mother in the grip of labor pain,
   To the baby with the heritage of sin,
To the cankered heirs of this our public stain,
   Does the Health Nurse bear the slogan that shall win.

To the suffering and needy and distressed
   Is she giving without stint her love and care;
And, wherever she is known, her name is blessed,
   And wherever she is needed, she is there.

So we'll doff our caps and help her when we can,
   As she goes about among the sick—and worse,
For she's doing what can not be done by man,
   She's a woman—and the Health Department Nurse.

AJPH 4 (December 1914): 1181.

23 "Ancient Occupation," 12.

24 See, for example, Lillian Wald, *Windows on Henry Street* (Boston: Little Brown, 1934), 75; Gardner, *Public Health Nursing*, 43–45; LaMotte, *Tuberculosis Nurse*, 88; and B. Franklin Royer, "Public Health Nursing vs. Bedside Nursing," *PHN* 15 (February 1923): 234.

25 Gardner, *Katharine Kent*, 66–67; and LaMotte, *Tuberculosis Nurse*, 88.

26 LaMotte, *Tuberculosis Nurse*, 88, 102–105.

27 The metaphor of seed and soil was the fashionable expression of this idea. "Hygiene and the Nurse," *Pacific Coast Journal of Nursing* 10 (January 1914): 157.

28 For example, in the case of the tuberculosis patient, the objective of the nurse was not so much to cure the disease but to prevent its spread to individuals not yet affected. LaMotte, *Tuberculosis Nurse*, 117; "Hygiene and the Nurse"; and Sir George Newman, "Preventive Medicine," *PHN* 12 (February 1920): 129–143.

29 "Hygiene and the Nurse," 57; Adelaide Nutting, "The Home and Its Relationship to Prevention of Disease," *AJN* 4 (September 1904): 913–924; Frankel, "Science and Public Health"; Winslow, "Untilled Field"; Eliot, "Main Points of Attack"; and Aikens, "Educational Opportunity."

30 "Hygiene and the Nurse." For a comparison with the views of Nightingale, see *Notes on Nursing*. See also Rosenberg, "Florence Nightingale," 116–136.

31 "Hygiene and the Nurse," 57. Hygiene was defined as the art of preserving health, of obtaining the most perfect action of body and mind "during as long a period as is consistent with the laws of life." Ibid. It aims at rendering growth more perfect, decay less rapid, life more vigorous, and death more remote.

32 Nutting, "Home," 117–118.

33 Ibid., 918–919.

34 Ibid.

35 LaMotte, *Tuberculosis Nurse*, 145.

36 Nutting, "Home," 918–919.

37 LaMotte, *Tuberculosis Nurse*, 148. While the basic message of the nurse was sunshine, good food, ventilation, and proper clothing, the exact details would of course vary with the needs of the specific patient. For example, the infant welfare nurse entered the homes of the poor, believing that at least one-half of all infant deaths were the result of ignorance on the part of the mother. Too many babies, claimed one worker in the field, "are ignorantly brought into the world; fed according to custom or fancy; treated when ill with much prejudice and superstition, doped with opium to 'cure colic'; suffocated in vitiated environments and stuffed with contaminated milk poorly modified." Having identified the problem, the work of the nurse seemed obvious; she would "open closed windows, remove superfluous clothes, prepare the baby's feeding, give it a bath and perform a hundred other services which together meant the difference between life and death." Richard Bolton, "Summer Work of the Baby Dispensary and Hospital of Cleveland," *VNQ* 2 (July 1910): 21; J. H. M. Knox, "The Opportunity of the Nurse in Reducing Infant Mortality," *VNQ* 2 (July 1910): 7–10; and H. J. Gerstenberger, "Babies Dispensary for Well Babies," *VNQ* 1 (April 1909): 24. For a detailed description of the care of the school-age child, see Florence Sherman, "Some Ways in Which Parents May Safeguard the Health of Their Children," *PHN* 11 (January 1919): 120–125.

38 Nutting, "Home," 917; and Annie Brainard, "The Visiting Nurse and Preventive Work," *VNQ* 1 (April 1909): 11. Ironically, having just written this comment, I heard a news report on the radio in which a Los Angeles health officer used these exact same words to describe his city's growing health problems that were the result of high rates of communicable disease among their immigrant population. National Public Radio, "All Things Considered," July 21, 1983.

39 Nutting, "Home," 917; and Lent, "True Functions," 577.

40 LaMotte, *Tuberculosis Nurse*, 18.

41 Ibid., 18–19. The best education was that which enabled the family to help them-selves. Mae Chamberlain, "How the Expectant Mother May Be Assisted by the Baby Health Station Service," *PHNQ* 10 (January 1918): 171.

42 Aikens, "Educational Opportunity," 186; LaMotte, *Tuberculosis Nurse*, 59, 218–223; Chamberlain, "Expectant Mother," 171; Lent, "True Functions," 578; and Wald, "Educational Value," 637.

43 Isabel Lowman, "A Morning with a Maternity Nurse," *VNQ* 1 (April 1909): 16–17.

44 Aikens, "Educational Opportunity," 186.

45 Ibid.; Chamberlain, "Expectant Mother," 171.

46 Aikens, "Educational Opportunity," 186–187, 189.

47 LaMotte, *Tuberculosis Nurse*, 2–3.

48 In a study of 2,020 tuberculosis patients, she found that only one-half of the patients were, as a result of the nurse's instructions, carefully following the techniques that had been taught to protect those around them, while the other half were classified as careless or grossly careless. The length of instruction seemed to have little effect on the outcomes, with those visited for over two years scoring only slightly higher than the patients seen for three months. LaMotte, *Tuberculosis Nurse*, 218–223.

49 Lent, "True Functions," 578.

50 Mary Lent, "Report of the Committee on Visiting Nursing," *AJN* 10 (June 1910): 866–868.

51 Ibid.

52 Wald, "Educational Value," 637.

53 Wald's idea of the school nurse was modeled after the English system. See Brain-ard, *Evolution*, 263–271; Lina Rogers, "What the Public School Nurse Is Doing," *VNQ* 2 (April 1910): 14–18; Lina Struthers (Rogers), *The School Nurse* (New York: Putnam, 1917); and Lavinia Dock, "The School Nurse Experiment in New York," *AJN* 3 (November 1902): 109–110.

54 Instructive District Nurse Association (IDNA) of Boston, *Annual Report* (1906), 19.

55 Nurses Report, IDNA of Boston, September 11, 1907.

56 Visiting Nurse Service (VNS) of Philadelphia, *Annual Report* (1904).

57 That year, $32,000 had been requested. VNS of Philadelphia, *Annual Report* (1906), 7.

58 Minutes of the Managers Meeting, VNS of Philadelphia, June 7, 1907; and Novem-ber 1907; and VNS of Philadelphia, *Annual Report* (1907), 6. In some cities, a slightly different plan evolved. In Chicago and Cleveland, for example, the board of health financed the school nurse program, while the Visiting Nurses Associa-tion provided the nurses and supervised their work. Brainard, *Evolution*, 230; and Waters, *Visiting Nursing*, 241.

59 Richard Shryock, *National Tuberculosis Association 1904–1954: A Study of the Voluntary Health Movement in the United States* (New York: National Tuberculosis Association, 1957), 47. Prior to 1900, there were probably only six sanatoriums in the United States; by 1910, this had increased to four hundred tuberculosis hospi-tals and sanatoriums.

60 Ibid., 28–29; the death rate for whites was 174 per 100,000 and for blacks was 485 per 100,000 in 1900. Shryock, *National Tuberculosis Association*, 64. Tuberculosis is described by many authors as a "house disease." See, for example, Edna Foley, "Home Teaching in Tuberculosis Cases," *TICTB* (1908): 539. William Osier appar-ently also used this description. See Brainard, *Evolution*, 274.

61 LaMotte, *Tuberculosis Nurse*, 275; Shryock, *National Tuberculosis Association*, 66; Sara Groves, "Instructive District Nurse Association: 1885–1912" (master's thesis,

Boston University, 1970), 69; and Nurses Report, IDNA of Boston, May/June 1908. According to the VNS of Philadelphia *Annual Report*, the work began in 1907, when they convinced the city to finance the work of the school nurse. At the time, only the Henry Phipps Institute sent "pupils" out to visit the tuberculosis patients attending their dispensary. The next year, the VNS added a second tuberculosis nurse and obtained money from the Pennsylvania Society for Prevention of Tuberculosis to conduct classes in a local church. The Pennsylvania Department of Health also opened its dispensary in Philadelphia that year with a staff of four nurses. Over the years, the state's program continued to grow, but their nurses provided only instructive services, leaving care of bedridden patients to the visiting nurse society. After 1919, the visiting nurse society discontinued having special tuberculosis nurses, and care for these patients was again provided by the general nursing staff. In 1923, the city health department took over the tuberculosis work from the state, and by 1930, there were twenty-nine city nurses and fourteen nurses from the Phipps Institute doing tuberculosis work. Although the VNS continued to take care of all bedside cases, as late as 1930, no plan had been developed to coordinate the work of these three organizations. VNS of Philadelphia, *Annual Report* (1907 and 1908); and the Minutes of the Managers Meeting, VNS of Philadelphia, June 16, 1919. See also Waters, *Visiting Nursing*, 264, 258; and Haven Emerson, *Philadelphia Hospital and Health Survey* (Philadelphia: Philadelphia Hospital and Health Survey Committee, 1930), 390–430, 442–445.

IDNA of Boston nurses started visiting tuberculosis patients in 1901, and by 1905, it had appointed its first special tuberculosis nurse. The special tuberculosis nurses did only educational and preventive work, while the regular staff provided any bedside care required by tuberculosis patients. IDNA had obtained special funds to support this work, apparently from the Society for the Relief and Control of Tuberculosis, but when they were discontinued in 1908, they concluded it was time for others to take over. Over time, tuberculosis nursing became the responsibility of the Boston Consumptive Hospital, Outpatient Department, which was the branch of municipal government responsible for tuberculosis patients in Boston. While the consumptive hospital and IDNA nurses both visited the bedridden advanced cases, they apparently never developed a very cooperative working relationship. IDNA of Boston, *Annual Report* (1906), 16; (1907), 7; and (1908), 14; Nurses Report, IDNA, May/June 1908; Waters, *Visiting Nursing*, 98–100, 325–326; and C.-E. A. Winslow et al., *The Community Health Association and Its Relationship to Boston's Health Program* (October 1926), Nursing Archive, n34, box 6, folder 2, pp. 8–10.

62 Irene Bower, *Public Health Nursing in Cleveland 1895–1928* (Cleveland: Western Reserve University, 1930), 63–71; and R. H. Bishop, "The Health Department," *VNQ* 3 (October 1911): 17.

Although Wald claims to have established, in 1893, the first systematic plan for instruction of the tuberculosis patient by visiting nurses, the work of Dr. and Mrs. William Osler in Baltimore is usually cited as the first organized effort of this kind. It was Lawrence Flick who first called attention to the dangers of "house infection." See William Olser, "The House in Its Relationship to the Tuberculosis Problem," *Medical News* 83 (December 1903): 1105–1110. Much as in Cleveland, the first tuberculosis dispensary was started by Dr. Osler at Hopkins, while Mrs. Osler raised money through private subscription to support the first tuberculosis nurse at the Visiting Nurse Association (VNA). Later, as the work grew, more nurses were added to the staff and their salaries were paid by the Maryland

Tuberculosis Association for Prevention of Tuberculosis. In 1910, the work of the nurses was taken over by the board of health. Wald, "Educational Value," 633; Water, *Visiting Nursing*, 92–94; and Brainard, *Evolution*, 273–279.

63 If Shryock's figures are correct, this represents a tremendous growth, since according to Wald, there were only 128 nurses employed by organizations doing only tuberculosis work and an additional 685 tuberculosis nurses on the staffs of visiting nurse societies in 1908. Shryock, *National Tuberculosis Association*, 119; and Wald, "Educational Value," 634.

64 Shryock, *National Tuberculosis Association*, 182–185. For the New York situation, see editorial, *AJN* 4 (February 1904): 410–411; Gloria Caliandro, "The Visiting Nurse in the Borough of Manhattan, New York City: 1877–1917" (EdD diss., Teachers' College, Columbia University, 1970), 113–128; Adelaide Nutting, "The Visiting Nurse for Tuberculosis," *Charities and the Commons* 16 (April 1906): 52; and Jane Delano, "Outline of Tuberculosis Work in Connection with Outpatient Department of Bellevue Hospital," *AJN* 4 (March 1904): 440–441. For Boston and Philadelphia, see note 49.

65 Shryock, *National Tuberculosis Association*, 118.

66 Caliandro, "Visiting Nurse," 113–128. The New York City Health Department was the first to hire visiting nurses to visit tuberculosis patients in 1903. As in most cities, these nurses' work was educational, and those patients requiring bedside care were referred to Henry Street Settlement or one of the other visiting nurse societies.

67 Ibid. See note 61 for Boston and Philadelphia.

68 Ibid.

69 Leavitt and Numbers, "Sickness and Health," 4, 7; and Davis, *Immigrant Health*, 58–59.

70 Rosen, *Preventive Medicine*, 47.

71 Brainard, *Evolution*, 282–304; Gardner, *Public Health Nursing*, 245–262; Knox, "Opportunity of the Nurse," 7–10; and Gerstenberger, "How to Start a Prophylactic Babies' Dispensary," 30–48.

72 Rosen, *Preventive Medicine*, 47.

73 VNS of Philadelphia, *Annual Report* (1911), 13.

74 Gardner, *Public Health Nursing*, 260.

75 Caliandro, "Visiting Nurse," 128–143.

76 VNS of Philadelphia, *Annual Report* (1906, 1908, and 1912); and Emerson, *Philadelphia Hospital and Health Survey*, 390, 412–416.

77 Bower, *PHN in Cleveland*, 71–75, 114.

78 Winslow, *Community Health Association*, 4, 12.

79 VNS of Philadelphia was given money in 1888 to "try out" an obstetrical nurse. In 1915, they decided to have their obstetrical nurse give prenatal care. Minutes of the Managers Meeting, VNS of Philadelphia, January 1888; May 1901; and May 7, 1915. The Providence District Nursing Association (DNA) began to visit patients discharged from the wards of Lying-in Hospital and Infants Wards of Rhode Island Hospital in 1911. DNA of Providence, *Annual Report* (1911), 31. Boston nurses started maternity work in 1901 when they formed a cooperative plan with the Boston Lying-In Hospital for the care of patients delivered at home by their externs. Between 1904 and 1914, Mrs. William Putnam funded a program in prenatal care. In addition, the obstetrical nurses visited patients from the Jewish Woman's Maternity Association and patients referred by an average of six hundred private physicians.

Mary Beard, *Instructive District Nursing Association: A Review* (Boston: September 1921), 15–20.

80   Joyce Antler and Daniel Fox, "The Movement toward a Safe Maternity: Physician Accountability in New York City, 1915–1940," *Bulletin of the History of Medicine* 50 (Winter 1976): 569–595; and J. Stanley Lemons, "The Sheppard-Towner Act: Progressivism in the 1920s," *Journal of American History* 55 (March 1969): 776–786.

81   For data related to the percent of maternity work being done by VNAs, see VNS of Philadelphia, *Annual Report* (1918), 8; and (1904), 11. For Boston, see IDNA of Boston, *Annual Report* (1909), 14–15; and Beard, "Review," 15–20, 25.

82   As early as 1931, a survey conducted by the National Organization for Public Health Nursing (NOPHN) confirmed that this was becoming the case nationwide.

Percentage of public health associations and departments of health carrying each of ten types of services

	PHN association	Dept. of health
Prenatal	100	72
Postpartum/neonatal	95	61
Health supv. infants	52	94
Health supv. preschooler	48	94
Morbidity / care of sick	95	28
Tuberculosis prevention	29	83
Delivery	38	—
School health	14*	66**
Communicable disease prevention	25	61
Syphilis/gonorrhea prevention	33	61

* PHN association providing school health where one nurse generalized programs in rural communities.

** All board of education nursing programs surveyed provided this service.

Committee on Field Studies and Administrative Practice of NOPHN, *Survey of Public Health Nursing: Administration and Practice* (New York: Commonwealth Fund, 1934), 152, 182, table 18.

83   DNA of Providence, *Annual Report* (1913), 30.

84   Goldmark, *Nursing and Nursing Education*, 42; and Waters, *Visiting Nursing*, 365.

85   In addition to the programs discussed, many associations initiated several smaller undertakings during this period. These included visiting housekeepers, visiting dieticians, programs for day nurseries, inspection of homes where children boarded, factory work, and programs for patients with contagious diseases.

86   These patterns of service delivery would continue until the passage of Medicare, at which time there was a dramatic increase in the number of local health departments offering services for the care of the sick. U.S. Department of Health, Education and Welfare, Public Health Service, Division of Nursing, *Services Available for Nursing Care of the Sick at Home*, January 1966, PHS Pub. No. 1256 (Revised 1967), 14.

87 For an example of this outcome, see Waters, *Visiting Nursing*, 315–377, where she lists in her statistical tables organizations employing visiting nurses by states and cities. By 1923, there were 121 national voluntary organizations: 22 were interested in the general promotion of health, 29 in specific diseases or health problems, and 70 only incidentally in promotion of health. John Ferrell, "The Trend of Preventive Medicine in the U.S.," *JAMA* 81 (September 1923): 1064.

88 As early as 1914, these discussions had occupied the attention of those attending the meetings of the American Public Health Association (APHA). See, for example, the series of articles "Relative Functions of Official and Non-official Health Agencies," *AJPH* 10 (December 1920): 940–972. In 1916, Gardner, in her just-published book on public health nursing, declared this issue one of the three major problems occupying the attention of those interested in the future of public health nursing. Gardner, *Public Health Nursing*, 56, 62–66.

89 Isabel Lowman, "Relationship of Private and Municipal Anti-tuberculosis Activities," *PHNQ* 6 (October 1914): 40–51.

90 Ibid. See also Charles Hatfield, "Relative Functions of Health Agencies: Viewpoint of the Non-official Agency," *AJPH* 10 (November 1920): 948–952; and John Ferrell, W. F. Snow, and Frederick Green, "Relative Functions of Health Agencies, Discussion," *AJPH* 10 (May 1920): 465–469.

91 Carl McCombs, "Public Health Departments and Private Health Agencies," *AJPH* 9 (December 1919): 951–955.

92 According to Curtis, this controversy between official and nonofficial agencies was not imaginary but actually occurring every day. France Curtis, "Relative Functions of Health Agencies: Relationship between Official and Non-official Agencies," *AJPH* 10 (January 1920): 956–960.

93 McCombs, "Public Health Departments."

94 Ibid., 955. See also Curtis, "Relative Functions."

95 McCombs, "Public Health Departments."

96 Emerson, "Meeting the Demand," 488.

97 Lavinia Dock, "The History of Public Health Nursing," *PHN* 14 (October 1922): 524.

98 Gardner, *Public Health Nursing*, 73.

99 Ira Wiles, "The Nurse of Tomorrow," *PHNQ* 7 (October 1915): 50. For the views of physicians, see also Harriet Leete, "Why Have Specialized Public Health Nurses?," *PHNQ* 8 (January 1916): 14–21; and "Various Opinions on General and Specialized Nursing," *PHNQ* 8 (January 1916): 56–59.

100 Annie Brainard, "The Many Sided Opportunity of Field Nursing," *PHNQ* 8 (January 1916): 52–55; and Austra Engel, "Specialization in Public Health Nursing," *PHNQ* 5 (October 19139): 36–41.

101 Brainard, "Opportunity of Field Nursing," 52–53. See, for example, DNA of Providence, *Annual Report* (1906–1907). Royer, "Public Health Nursing."

102 Brainard, "Opportunity of Field Nursing." Public health nurses often mentioned this distinction between working with one's hands versus one's mind. See, for example, Mary Gardner, "The Changing Emphasis in Public Health Nursing," *Proceedings for the International Congress of Nurses* (January 1926): 47; and Editorial, "The Youngest Professional," *VNQ* 3 (April 1911): 6. For the public health nurse, like so many other groups aspiring for professional status, the greatest prestige was assigned to those activities that removed her form what Andrew Abbott, in a recent article on professional status, called the "front lines." Andrew Abbott, "Status and Status Strain in the Professions," *American Journal of Sociology* 86 (January 1981):

819–835. For a discussion on these ideas in terms of women in the professions, see Joan Jacobs Brumberg and Nancy Tomes, "Women in the Professions: A Research Agenda for American Historians," *Reviews in American History* 10 (June 1982): 276–289.

103 Wiles, "Nurse of Tomorrow," 50.

104 Engel, "Specialization."

105 Rosenkrantz, "Cart before Horse," and *Public Health and the State*, especially chapters 4 and 5; George Rosen, *The Structure of American Medical Practice, 1875–1941* (Philadelphia: University of Pennsylvania Press, 1983), 40–43; and John Duffy, "The American Medical Profession and Public Health: From Support to Ambivalence," *Bulletin of the History of Medicine* 53 (Spring 1979): 1–22.

106 S. Josephine Baker, "Generalized versus Specialized Nursing," *PHNQ* 8 (January 1916): 40–42; H. W. Hill, "Is the Visiting Nurse a Public Health Nurse?," *PHN* 11 (July 1919): 486–488; and Royer, "Public Health Nursing."

107 Elizabeth Fox, "Is a Visiting Nurse a Public Health Nurse?," *PHN* 11 (July 1919): 575–577; Editorial, "Theory or Experience," *PHN* 11 (July 1919): 579–581; Lee Frankel, "Is the Visiting Nurse a Public Health Nurse?," *PHN* 11 (July 1919): 698–702; and "A Letter from a Visiting Nurse," *PHN* 11 (September 1919): 703. In response to the editor's request, numerous nurses wrote to the *PHN*, confirming the editor's belief that "the visiting nurse is fundamentally a public health nurse." "Conclusion," *PHN* 11 (September 1919): 703.

108 The visiting nurse would not, like these specialists, become a scientist and teacher at the expense of tender ministrations. Brainard, "Evolution," 420; Editorial, "Further Opportunities for Visiting Nursing," *PHNQ* 7 (January 1915): 16–18; Harriet Fulmer, "The Pioneers in Public Health Nursing," *PHNQ* 7 (January 1915): 19–22; and Editorial, "Theory or Experience," 579.

109 Gardner, herself probably the only superintendent of a large VNA that supported specialization, reviews the arguments of the critics. Gardner, *Public Health Nursing*, 579.

110 Beard, "Generalization," 42–47; Mary Mackenzie, "District Nurse," *PHNQ* 7 (January 1915): 29–34; and Lillian Wald to Adelaide Nutting, May 1911, Nursing Archives, Teachers College, Columbia.

111 Beard, "Generalization."

112 Edna Foley, "The Past and Future of Tuberculosis Nurses," in *The National Association for the Study and Prevention of Tuberculosis: Transactions of the Seventh Annual Meeting* (Philadelphia: WM. F. Fell, 1911), 122; Winslow, "New Profession"; Beard, "Generalization"; and Bessie LeLacheur, "The General Visiting Nurse," *PHNQ* 7 (January 1915): 23–26. Wald was vigorously opposed to "over-specialization." See, for example, Lillian Wald to Lee Frankel, May 9, 1913, Wald Collection, box 2, roll 1, folder 1913; and Lillian Wald to Elizabeth Crawell, October 21, 1912, Wald Collection, box 2, roll 1, folder 1912.

113 See, for example, the February 1923 issue of the *PHN*, which is devoted to this issue.

114 This debate resulted in a major demonstration project as well as a national study. Although both supported the idea of "generalization," neither produced the desired outcome, and visiting nurses continued to care for the sick, while the nurses at the health departments taught the well. East Harlem Nursing and Health Service, *Comparative Study*; and Goldmark, *Nursing and Nursing Education*. For the long-range outcome, see note 82. Strong supporters of this idea were the advocates of

the neighborhood health center movement. For a discussion of this movement, see George Rosen, "The First Neighborhood Health Center Movement: Its Rise and Fall," *AJPH* 61 (August 1971): 1620–1635.

Chapter 4 — Preserving the Treasures of Their Tradition

1   Lillian Wald to Mrs. Whitelaw Reid, December 2, 1913, in *History of American Red Cross Nursing*, ed. Lavinia Dock et al. (New York: Macmillan, 1922), 1220.

2   Mary Gardner to Ella Crandall, December 29, 1911, Gardner Papers, folder 45.

3   As early as 1893, the need for some kind of national organization had been publicly discussed. See, for example, Somerville, "District Nursing," in *Nursing of the Sick*, 126. The idea of a federation of visiting nurses was also discussed at the 1904 meeting of the National Conference of Charities and Corrections. The visiting nurses in attendance decided that "for the present this would not be advisable," planning instead to meet yearly as a group in connection with this conference. The first national conference of visiting nurses was held in April 1908 at the suggestion of the Chicago Visiting Nurse Association (VNA), with 108 nurses attending. See Anne Doyle, untitled paper on the origins of the National Organization for Public Health Nursing (NOPHN), 1937, Gardner Papers, folder 45, pp. 2–8.

4   Isabel Lowman, "The Need of a Standard for Visiting Nursing," *VNQ* 4 (January 1912): 14.

5   For a detailed description of the Metropolitan Life Insurance Company (MLI) situation, see Crandall, "Memoranda." The company's service had been organized in 1909 as a strictly graduate nurse program in accordance with the standards for the work stipulated by Wald. Crandall had organized the nursing service for MLI before becoming an instructor at Teachers College, Columbia. Eleanor Mumford, "Field Interview with Ella Phillips Crandall," January 19, 1937, Gardner Papers, folder 45. In one of the associations approached by Frankel, the company had paid for 33,494 visits that year. See Allison, "Shall Attendants Be Trained and Registered?," 933.

6   Wald, Foley, and Crandall discussed the matter with Frankel, reminding him of the terms and conditions stipulated by Wald when the service was initiated. To these nurses, the company's action seemed to indicate a serious tendency toward commercialism. Crandall, "Memoranda."

7   Edna Foley, "Concerning the Employing of Practical Nurses by Visiting Nurse Associations," *AJN* 12 (January 1912): 328, 330.

8   Annie Goodrich, "The Need for Orientation," *AJN* 13 (February 1913): 341.

9   After initiating this program around 1913, the company was able to reduce the number of visits to chronic cases by over twenty thousand each year. MLI, *Work of Metropolitan Life Insurance*, 3.

10 Lowman, "Need of a Standard."

11 Committee members from the American Nurses' Association were Delano, Anna Kerr, and Crandall; from the Superintendents Society, they were Foley, Gardner, and Beard. All were public health nurses. See "Report of the Joint Committee Appointed for Consideration of the Standardization Visiting Nursing," in *Proceedings of the Eighteenth Annual Convention of the American Society of Superintendents of Training Schools for Nurses* (Springfield, Mass.: Thatcher Art Printery, 1912), 118–124. See also the discussion of establishment of NOPHN in Fitzpatrick, *National Organization*, 20–36; and Brainard, *Evolution*, 323–344.

12 Doyle, untitled paper, p. 8.

13 Ibid, pp. 8–10; and Brainard, *Evolution*, 329–330.

14 Doyle, untitled paper, pp. 10–13.

15 "The 15th National Convention of the American Nurses Association," *VNQ* 4 (July 1912): 43–68.

16 "Constitution of the NOPHN," article 2, 1912, Wald Collection.

17 Brainard, *Evolution*, 334. The discussion leading to this decision is presented in "15th National Convention."

18 Doyle, untitled paper, pp. 12–14; and Fitzpatrick, *National Organization*, 23–25.

19 Wald was elected president; Foley, vice president; Crandall, secretary; and Lent, treasurer. The following were elected to the first board of directors: Beard, superintendent, Instructive District Nursing Association (IDNA), Boston; Delano, chairman, National Committee, Red Cross Nursing Service; Gardner, superintendent, District Nursing Association (DNA) of Providence; Flora Glen, superintendent of nurses, Municipal Tuberculosis Sanitarium, Chicago; Anne L. Hansen, domestic educator, Immigrants League of Buffalo; Sarah B. Helbert, School Nurse for the Cincinnati Anti-Tuberculosis League; Edith M. Hickey, school nurse, Seattle, Washington; Lydia A. Hollman, superintendent, Holman Association, Alta Pass, North Carolina; Matilda Johnson, superintendent, VNA of Cleveland; Anna W. Kerr, superintendent of School Nurses, New York City Department of Health; Ellen La Motte, superintendent of Tuberculosis Nurses of Baltimore; Harriet L. Leet, superintendent of Nurses, Babies Dispensary and Hospital of Cleveland; Minnie Patterson, superintendent, VNA of Minneapolis; and Julia C. Stimson, head worker, Social Service Department, Washington University Hospital, St. Louis. Fitzpatrick, *National Organization*, 26.

20 Isabel Lowman, "The National Seal for the Visiting Nurse Association," *AJN* 8 (June 1908): 715–717; "A Common Seal," *VNQ* 2 (January 1910): 6–9; and Fitzpatrick, *National Organization*, 27. The emblem symbolized "the implanting in the hearts and minds of the sick poor the desire for better, cleaner, higher living that will enable them to work toward their own rescue from the unfortunate conditions which hold them back from happier times." "15th National Convention," 62–63.

21 "15th National Convention," 62; and Fitzpatrick, *National Organization*, 27.

22 "15th National Convention," 62. According to Louise Fitzpatrick, the board's first choice for executive secretary was Delano, but she refused the position. Crandall was the choice of Wald. Fitzpatrick, *National Organization*, 29–30.

23 Ella Crandall to Jane Delano, January 3, 1913, Red Cross Collection; and Miss Crandall, untitled circular letter to the readers of the *Quarterly*, disapproving of Dr. Frankel's plan, National Archives Gift Collection, RG 200, Records of American National Red Cross, 1886–1916, box 40, folder 500.002, MLI.

24 Ibid.

25 Crandall, "Memorandum."

26 Frankel was so eager to discuss his proposal with the executive committee that he offered to pay their way to New York at their earliest convenience. Crandall eventually convinced him to postpone this discussion until the convention. Ella Crandall to Jane Delano, January 11, 1913, Red Cross Collection.

27 Mary Beard, "Address," in *Proceedings of the Twenty-Third Annual Convention of the National League of Nursing Education* (Baltimore, Md.: Williams & Wilkins, 1917), 61.

28 Frankel, "Visiting Nursing," 25–45. The reaction to Frankel's paper is discussed further in chapter 2.

29　"Report of the Executive Committee of NOPHN, June 21–27, 1913," Wald Collection, roll 31.

30　Frankel's concerns were next discussed at the June 25, 1915, board of directors meeting. Although "the secretary [Ella Crandall] was instructed to continue to urge, by all possible means, the establishment of a fee system as a matter of principle, 'little materially changed.'" Minutes of the Board of Directors Meeting, June 25, 1915, NOPHN Collection, National League for Nursing, New York (hereafter cited as NOPHN Collection), roll 11. Cleveland initiated a two year trial study of "hourly nursing," probably in response to Frankel's concerns, the same year. Minutes of the Executive Committee Meeting of NOPHN, January 18–20, 1915, Wald Collection, roll 31. Crandall also wrote an article in support of "hourly nursing" (i.e., fee-for-service care for pay patients on an hourly basis), where she suggests that no other single factor would so quickly and effectively lift the "stigma of charity" that rests on VNAs. Ella Crandall, "Care of the Sick in Their Homes," *PHNQ* 7 (January 1915): 13.

31　Patterson, "First Annual Meeting," 13.

32　Editorial, "The Atlantic City Meeting," 5–7; Ella Crandall, "The National Organization for Public Health Nursing and Its Relationship to Local Societies," *PHNQ* 5 (January 1913): 11–19; and Lillian Wald, "Presidential Address," *PHNQ* 5 (1912): 21–29.

33　Elizabeth Fox, "One Visiting Nurse's Impression of the Conference," *PHNQ* 6 (July 1914): 14. According to Mrs. Codman, only ten lady managers attended the convention. Although the managers were in the minority, "the nurses did everything they could to make us feel as if we were professionals." IDNA of Boston, *Annual Report* (1913), 17; and "Report of the Two Informal Meetings of the Visiting Nurse Managers," IDNA Collection, n34, box 2, folder 6.

34　Patterson, "First Annual Meeting," 13.

35　Mary Gardner, "President's Address," *PHNQ* 6 (July 1914): 20–23.

36　Mary Gardner, "President's Address, Third Annual Meeting, NOPHN," *PHNQ* 7 (October 1915): 29–33.

37　Approximately ninety-six people attended the convention: fifty members, twenty-six delegates, and twenty guests. Winifred Fitzpatrick, "Report of the Meeting of NOPHN," *PHNQ* 7 (October 1915): 16; "Statement from the NOPHN, December 10, 1920," Winslow Collection, 87:1391; and Mrs. Ireland to Ella Crandall, [about 1913], NOPHN Collection, roll 25.

38　Minutes of the Mid-year Meeting, Executive Committee of NOPHN, January 18–20, 1915, IDNA Collection, n34, box 2, folder 6, pp. 7–9.

39　Ibid., pp. 9–11.

40　Ibid., pp. 8, 11.

41　Ibid., pp. 9–10.

42　Ibid., p. 10; and Minutes of the Advisory Council of NOPHN, March 22, 1915, NOPHN Collection, roll 26, pp. 10, 12.

43　Ibid.

44　"Source Material," vol. 8, Rockefeller Foundation Archives (hereafter cited as RF Archives), pp. 2077–2079. Crandall wrote to Mr. John D. Rockefeller on October 13, 1914; Rose wrote to Greene of his decision on July 30, 1915, but Crandall was not told of their final decision until November 11, 1915.

45　"The Secretary's Third Annual Report, 1916," NOPHN Collection, roll 27.

46　"The Fourth Annual Report of NOPHN," *PHNQ* 8 (July 1916): 11–12, 17.

47   Ibid., 20–21. Frankel suggested that a special committee be immediately appointed to consider these needs. A year later, Katharine Codman, a member of the IDNA of Boston board, was appointed chairman of such a committee. "Report of the Committee on Organization and Administration, December 31, 1917 and June 14, 1918," NOPHN Collection, roll 25. Ironically, Codman was the wife of Ernest Amory Codman, a Boston surgeon whose passion for evaluating medical intervention in terms of "end results" had by 1915 resulted in his forced resignation from the medical society, the loss of his teaching position at Harvard, and financial disaster. See Susan Reverby, "Stealing the Golden Eggs: Ernest Amory Codman and the Science and Management of Medicine," *Bulletin of the History of Medicine* 55 (Summer 1981): 156–171. Although Mrs. Codman's committee had expansive plans, by 1919, they had accomplished little. In fact, it was not until 1922, when the MLI provided a $15,000 budget, that the NOPHN began to seriously address the issue of evaluation. See "Resolution Adopted at the Business Meeting, NOPHN, July 1, 1922," NOPHN Collection, roll 11; and "Report of the Executive Committee, September 18–19, 1922," NOPHN Collection, roll 11. The study was completed in 1924. Minutes of the Board of Directors Meeting, NOPHN Meeting, June 21, 1924, NOPHN Collection, roll 11.

48   "Fourth Annual Report," 10–11.

49   Dock, *Red Cross*, 1220.

50   The nurses involved in the early development of the Red Cross Rural Nursing Service were Wald, Delano, Goodrich, Fox, Clements, and Gardner. See, for example, Dock, *Red Cross*, 1211–1215; and Portia B. Kernodle, *The Red Cross Nurse in Action, 1882–1948* (New York: Harper, 1949), 69–71.

51   Mary Beard to Mrs. Codman, April 4, 1912, IDNA Collection, n34, box 1, folder 4. In her letter of December 2, 1913, Wald mentions that the same people are interested in both the NOPHN and the Rural Nursing Service. Dock, *Red Cross*, 1220.

52   Fox makes reference to the shifting attention of the leaders of American affairs from city life to country life in "Red Cross Public Health Nursing," *PHN* 12 (February 1920): 175. See also Fannie Clements, "Rural Nursing," *AJN* 13 (February 1913): 370.

53   Kernodle, *Red Cross Nurse*, 70–71. Jane Delano, "The Red Cross," *AJN* 13 (January 1913): 281.

54   Dock, *Red Cross*, 1214; and Kernodle, *Red Cross Nurse*, 70–72.

55   Schiff provided $5,000 and Reid $1,000 to finance a trial year. If successful, Schiff also promised to establish a $100,000 endowment to be used by the service, plus $5,000 a year until the service was permanently established. Reid later increased her annual contribution to $2,000. Dock, *Red Cross*, 1215.

56   Kernodle, *Red Cross Nurse*, 41; and Dock, *Red Cross*, 25, 47, 1216.

57   Dock, *Red Cross*, 1216–1217; and Brainard, *Evolution*, 301. They also tried to avoid the stigmatizing of "charity image" that plagued many VNAs from the onset by establishing that "as a rule, patients are expected to pay for professional visits according to their means, but those unable to do so should not go uncared for." Fannie Clements, "Rural Nursing," *AJN* 13 (April 1913): 521.

58   Kernodle, *Red Cross Nurse*, 73; Dock, *Red Cross*, 1235; and Jane Delano, "The Red Cross," *AJN* 13 (April 1913): 281.

59   Clements, "Rural Nursing," 521. Prior to World War I, organization of the Red Cross by chapters was only slightly developed. The strongest chapters were in large

cities, and few took up "health conservation" work. Only after the United States' entry into World War I did the rural chapters begin to organize, but they failed to show interest in public health nursing until after the war. Dock, *Red Cross*, 1271. Dock lists the early affiliation (1913–1914) that represented a wide variety of organizations ranging from VNAs to mutual aid societies, health leagues, and industry. Dock, *Red Cross*, 1269–1270.

60 Kernodle, *Red Cross Nurse*, 73–74; and Dock, *Red Cross*, 1218. In her survey of the forty visiting nurse societies employing more than three nurses, Clements found that only six offered a course; most were only three months long and included little classroom instruction. They included IDNA of Boston, Henry Street Settlement, and visiting nurse societies of Chicago; Detroit; Richmond; Buffalo; Concord, New Hampshire; and Orange, New Jersey. The first Red Cross Scholarship students were sent to IDNA of Boston for a four-month course.

61 Westchester County DNA was the first rural nursing service organized in the United States. Its program was initiated in 1912 with six nurses serving twenty villages. Kernodle, *Red Cross Nurse*, 69. Dock discusses the impact of the Red Cross standards and scholarships on the development of public health nursing education. Dock, *Red Cross*, 1235–1255. For the Teachers College program, see Marshall, *Mary Adelaide Nutting*, 206.

62 Kernodle, *Red Cross Nurse*, 73–74. Abbie Roberts was appointed supervisor. She was a graduate of Jewish Hospital of Cincinnati, had experience in infant welfare and tuberculosis work with the board of health, spent ten months at Henry Street Settlement, and helped to organize the VNA of Cincinnati for four years. She had just completed the rural nursing course at Teachers College prior to joining the Red Cross staff. Requirements for appointment, duties, vacation (thirty days/year), and salary ($60/month) are described in Fannie Clements, "American Red Cross Town and Country Nursing Service," *AJN* 14 (May 1914): 540; and Jane Delano, "The Red Cross," *AJN* 14 (January 1914): 285.

63 Dock, *Red Cross*, 1219.

64 Ibid., 1226; Kernodle, *Red Cross Nurse.*, 75; and "Executive Committee Meeting NOPHN, 21–27 June 1913," Wald Collection, Record group NOPHN, roll 31.

65 Lillian Wald to Mrs. Whitelaw Reid, December 2, 1913. In Dock, *Red Cross*, 1220.

66 Dock, *Red Cross*, 1220–1221. Boardman was apparently a strong advocate of a rapidly expanding nursing service. Clements believed such rapid growth would mean abandoning their position on special preparation for rural nursing and resisted rapid growth. Boardman also pushed the Red Cross to establish its own teaching centers large enough to accommodate thirty to forty nurses. Kernodle, *Red Cross Nurse*, 76–77, 86.

67 Dock, *Red Cross*, 1221. In March 1915, a town was defined as twenty-five thousand people. Reid resigned as chair of the Town and Country Nursing Service Committee, shifting her financial support and interest to foreign relief activities. She was replaced by Mrs. Harriet Blaine Beale, for many years associated with the Visiting Nurse Society (VNS) of Washington, DC. Dock, *Red Cross*, 1234–1264.

68 Kernodle, *Red Cross Nurse*, 77, 82–85; and Dock, *Red Cross*, 1291–1292. These percentages are for 1916, at which time there were sixty-six nurses who cared for 10,286 patients, providing a total of 112,836 visits. All but one of these nurses worked in a town of five hundred to ten thousand people. Their visiting area varied, depending on the number of people served, but ranged from two to eight square miles.

Comparing Red Cross nurses to Boston IDNA nurses for a similar year

	IDNA	Red Cross
Staff	59	66
Patients	20,769	10,286
Visits	128,742	112,836
Patients/Nurse	3,520	155
Visits/Nurse	2,182	1,709
Visits/Patient	6.2	11

Not surprisingly, the Red Cross nurses cared for fewer patients and made fewer visits than the city nurses but interestingly made, on the average, more visits to each patient. IDNA of Boston, *Annual Report* (1917).

69   For a discussion of the NOPHN and Red Cross relations during World War I, see Fitzpatrick, *National Organization*, 44–82. The issue of sending nurses to Europe was discussed at the January 18–20, 1915, executive committee meeting. Prior to the meeting, all directors' and officers' opinions had been polled on this issue of the Red Cross's sending nurses to Europe: twelve approved, one had resigned, one was away, one did not reply, thirty were opposed, and the resident was ill. Despite the apparent agreement, Delano was able to convince those attending the meeting to drop the matter. Minutes of the Mid-year Meeting, Executive Committee of NOPHN, January 18–20, 1915, IDNA Collection, n34, box 2, folder 6, pp. 6–7.

70   Minutes of the Mid-year Meeting, pp. 6–7.

71   These included Beard, Gardner, Waters, Lent, and "various others," according to Crandall. Ella Crandall to C.-E. A. Winslow, April 19, 1917, Winslow Collection, 86:1389.

72   Ibid. One of their major concerns was the lack of adequate supervision. This was an apparently newly acquired attitude, for as late as March 1915, the advisory council had discussed amalgamation of the NOPHN with the Red Cross as a plausible solution to their "overlapping" purposes. Minutes of the Advisory Council of NOPHN, March 22, 1915, NOPHN Collection, roll 26.

73   Delano's proposal is discussed in a letter from C.-E. A. Winslow to the members of the advisory council, April 19, 1917, Winslow Collection, 86:1389.

74   Minutes of the Advisory Council of NOPHN, April 10, 1917, Winslow Collection, 87:1413.

75   "A Statement of the Field and Function of the NOPHN," Winslow Collection, 86:1384.

76   Kernodle, *Red Cross Nurse*, 121.

77   Mary Beard, "Address," 59–63.

78   Minutes of the Board of Directors Meeting of the NOPHN, May 2, 1917; and Minutes of the Advisory Council of NOPHN, May 4, 1917, NOPHN Collection, roll 11.

79   Mary Beard, "President's Address to the NOPHN," *PHNQ* 9 (July 1917): 213.

80   J. Stanley Lemon, *The Woman Citizen: Social Feminism in the 1920s* (Chicago: University of Illinois Press, 1973), 5–20.

81   "Fifth Annual Report of the Executive Secretary, April, 1917," NOPHN Collection, roll 11.

82   Crandall's letter was discussed at the April 3, 1917, Meeting of the Managers, VNS of Philadelphia.

83 After the Red Cross turned down their request, the NOPHN initially planned to take no further action. But at the meeting of the advisory council (May 2, 1917) following the convention, this decision was reversed. Minutes of the Advisory Council of NOPHN, May 2–4, 1917, NOPHN Collection, roll 11.

84 Ella Crandall to C.-E. A. Winslow, May 15, 1917, Winslow Collection, 86:1389; and Minutes of the Advisory Council, June 4, 1917, Winslow Collection, 100:1764–1766.

85 Beard was given a leave of absence from the IDNA of Boston to work full time in these and other NOPHN-related activities. Fitzpatrick, *National Organization*, 59. For a description of the work of Beard's committee, see "The Three Nursing Committees of the Council of National Defense," *PHNQ* 9 (October 1917): 319, 329. The members included Gardner, Delano, Colonel Henry Birmingham, Mrs. John Higbee, Dr. John Fulton, Assistant Surgeon General Stimpson, and Ella Crandall.

86 Apparently, Colonel Means opposed "the pronouncement." Minutes of the Advisory Council of NOPHN, July 8, 1917, NOPHN Collection, roll 11.

87 The committee's work was initiated by Wald, Nutting, Crandall, Stewart, and Goodrich in the spring of 1917. Their first meeting was June 4, 1917, and by June 6, they had announced their full membership. Marshall, *Mary Adelaide Nutting*, 223–228. For an excellent discussion of the role of professional nurses in the war and the difficulties they encountered and their very different (from public health nurses) relationship with laywomen, see Susan Armeny, "Organized Nurses, Women Philanthropists and the Intellectual Bases for Cooperation among Women, 1898–1920," in *Nursing History: New Perspectives. New Possibilities*, ed. Ellen Lagenman (New York: Teachers College Press, 1983), 13–45; and Nancy Tomes, "A Collision of Nursing's Two Worlds: Volunteer and Professional Nurses in World War I" (paper presentation, Fifth Berkshire Conference on the History of Women, June 18, 1981).

88 "Three Nursing Committees," 329.

89 Ibid., 318. "Report of the Board of Directors and Advisory Council of the NOPHN, July 23, 1917," Winslow Collection, 100:1764, p. 4.

90 Brainard, *Evolution*, 347; Marshall, *Nutting*, 227; and Fitzpatrick, *National Organization*, 60–61.

91 Report of the NOPHN, July 23, 1917.

92 Ibid., 4. "Annual Report of the NOPHN January 1, 1918–January 1, 1919," NOPHN Collection, roll 25.

93 Lent's activities are described in the following: Mary Lent, "Public Health Nursing in the Extra-cantonment Zone," *AJPH* 9 (May 1919): 193–195; Mary Lent, "Public Health Nursing in the Extra-containment Zones," *PHNQ* 10 (July 1918): 264–275; assistant surgeon general D. S. Warren, "Unified Health Service," *PHN* 11 (July 1919): 489–492; Mary Lent, "Sanitary Conditions about Military Camps and Parts Played by Public Health Nurses," in *Proceedings of the National Conference of Social Work at the Forty-Fifth Annual Session* (Chicago: Rogers & Hall, 1918), 189; and Annie Brainard, "The Extra-cantonment Sanitary Zones," *PHNQ* 10 (January 1918): 7–17.

94 "Annual Report of the Executive Secretary, December 1916–December 1917," NOPHN Collection, roll 11.

95 Beard simply sought financial assistance, but Dr. Vincent apparently had something grander in mind for the NOPHN. As a result of their conversation, Vincent concluded that the NOPHN should move to Baltimore and establish an alliance with the new School of Hygiene and Public Health that the foundation was supporting

at the Johns Hopkins University. The idea appealed to both Beard and Vincent, and they agreed to meet again for further discussion. Vincent's enthusiasm was not shared by the other officers of the foundation. Vincent, still hoping to establish some relationship between the two organizations, even if "of a less intimate sort," arranged a luncheon conference to that end among Beard, Flexner, and Welch. In the end, the proposal was abandoned. History 900–902, "Source Material," vol. 8, RF Archives, pp. 2079–2082.

96   NOPHN 1914–1917, RF Archives, 200C-box 121, Old 1498.

97   "The Chicago Meeting of the NOPHN," *PHN* 11 (January 1919): 152.

98   VNS of Philadelphia, *Annual Report* (1918), 11.

99   In 1917, each nurse cared for 296 patients, making 9.4 visits/patient, while in 1918, each cared for 316 patients, making 7.9 visits/patient. Despite the increase in annual budget, the Boston association's deficit remained stable at $2,000/year. IDNA of Boston, *Annual Report* (1917), 23; and (1918), 39. In Providence, the number of patients cared for increased from 8,390 in 1917 to 10,332 in 1918, while the number of visits/patient decreased from 12.7 to 10.2. DNA of Providence, *Annual Reports* (1917), 15; and (1918), 17.

100   IDNA of Boston, *Annual Report* (1918), 12; and DNA of Providence, *Annual Report* (1919), 8.

101   Philadelphia lost twelve staff, Providence lost fourteen nurses (out of forty-six), and Boston lost eight to "war service." VNS of Philadelphia, *Annual Report* (1918), 11; DNA of Providence, *Annual Report* (1918), 24; and IDNA of Boston, *Annual Report* (1918), 21.

102   DNA of Providence, *Annual Report* (1919), 8.

103   Minutes of the Managers Meeting, VNS of Philadelphia, April 18, 1918. Boston, for example, the same year had seven staff resign to go to "other" positions; only one less than the number going with the Red Cross. IDNA of Boston, *Annual Report* (1918), 21.

104   Minutes of the Managers Meeting, VNS of Philadelphia, April 18, 1918.

105   Minutes of the Managers Meeting, VNS of Philadelphia, June 2, 1917; and VNS of Philadelphia, *Annual Report* (1917), 17.

106   VNS of Philadelphia, *Annual Report* (1917), 13; and Minutes of the Supervisors Meeting, IDNA of Boston, June 3, 1918; and August 9, 1918.

107   Minutes of the Managers Meeting, VNS of Philadelphia, June 2, 1917.

108   "Executive Committee of the NOPHN, June 4, 1917," NOPHN Collection, roll 11.

109   "Executive Committee of the NOPHN, December 14–16, 1917," NOPHN Collection, roll 11. An attendant service was initiated as an experiment by the Cleveland VNA in March 1915. Its outcome is discussed in Blanche Swainhart, "The Supervised Attendant Service," in *Proceedings of the Twenty-Fourth Annual Convention of the National League of Nursing Education* (Baltimore, Md.: Williams & Wilkins, 1919), 195–217.

110   This was not an original solution. Emerson's new worker was modeled after the role of the English health visitor. S. O. Baker to Haven Emerson, December 17, 1918, Nutting Papers, "health visitor" folder, Teachers College, Columbia University, New York (hereafter cited as MAN Collection).

111   See the letters written by nursing leadership in response to Emerson's proposal in the "health visitor" folder, MAN Collection. The Emerson quotation can be found in Haven Emerson to M. Nutting, August 1, 1917, "health visitor" folder, MAN Collection. The new role and salary are discussed in M. Adelaide Nutting,

"Memorandum on Training for Health Visitors, July 13, 1917," "health visitor" folder, MAN Collection. To put the smallness of this salary into perspective, it should be noted that in 1909, the health department was paying nurses $900–$1,200/year. Waters, *Visiting Nursing*, 341.

112 J. A. Duffy, *A History of Public Health in New York City: 1866–1966* (New York: Russell Sage, 1974), 276, mentions his removal from office. For a more detailed discussion of these various plans, see E. V. Brumbaugh, "Public Health Instructor—a New Type of Health Worker," *AJPH* 18 (September 1918): 662–664; Agnes Randolph, "The New Law in Virginia," *PHNQ* 10 (July 1918): 295–301; and Kernodle, *Red Cross Nurse*, 166–178.

113 Minutes of the Advisory Council of NOPHN, November 11, 1918, Winslow Collection, 87:1413.

114 Robertson presented his plan in John Dill Robertson, "Who Shall Nurse the Sick?," *AJPH* 11 (January 1921): 108–112. The story of the nurse is quoted from Amy Hillard, "A Discussion of the Report of the Rockefeller Committee and Its Effect in Practice upon the Hospital Nursing Department," in *Transactions of the American Hospital Association: Twenty-Fourth Annual Conference* (Chicago: American Hospital Association, 1922), 182.

115 Randolph, "New Law in Virginia," 296. Vincent's views are discussed in a letter from Ella Crandall to C.-E. A. Winslow, November 21, 1918, Winslow Collection, 86:1390.
    See also Fitzpatrick, *National Organization*, 72–76; and T. E. Christy et al., "An Appraisal of 'An Abstract for Action,'" in *A Source Book of Nursing Research*, ed. Florence Downs and Margaret Newman (Philadelphia: F. A. Davis, 1973), 230.

116 Randolph, "New Law in Virginia," 297.

117 M. Grace O'Brien, "Training, Licensure and Supervision of Attendants," in *Proceedings of the Twenty-Fourth Annual Convention*, 222; and "Code for Aid and Attendant Service under Public Health Nursing Agencies," *PHNQ* 10 (July 1918): 302. See also Fitzpatrick, *National Organization*, 302; Mary Beard, "The Attendant as an Assistant to the Public Health Nurse," *PHN* 11 (March 1919): 181–183; Florence Caldwell, "The Attendant as an Assistant to Public Health Nurses," *PHN* 11 (May 1919): 346; Dorothy Deming, *The Practical Nurse* (New York: Commonwealth Fund, 1947), 184; and Blanche Swainhart, "The Supervised Attendant Service," *PHNQ* 10 (April 1918): 183–198.

118 "Business Meeting of the NOPHN, May 10, 1918," NOPHN Collection, roll 35. At the same meeting, the members discussed the use of "unqualified graduate nurses or other persons" to assist the staff during the war. They decided to call unqualified graduate nurses substitutes, and partially trained attendants and aids would be called emergency assistants.

119 Mary Beard to the Women's Committee, Council for National Defense, July 3, 1918, Winslow Collection, 100:1766, pp. 2–4.

120 For more details, see Tomes, "Nursing's Two Worlds"; and Armery, "Organized Nurses, Women Philanthropists."

121 Chester Bolton was an aide to the assistant secretary of war. Bolton's activities are described in David Loth, *A Long Way Forward: The Biography of Congresswoman Frances P. Bolton* (New York: Longmans, Green, 1957), 89–111.

122 "Executive Secretary's Report, NOPHN, December 1916–December 1917," NOPHN Collection, roll 25. The committee was formed in fall 1917. Its name was changed to War Program Committee in recognition of its larger "possibilities." Part of the

committee's charge was to increase the membership of the NOPHN and therefore increase its income, but it had minimal success.

"Statement from the NOPHN, December 10, 1920."

	NOPHN Disbursements	Amount from Membership	%
1917	$22,553	$3,472	15
1918	42,792	5,280	10
1919	81,501	6,449	7.9

Winslow Collection, 87:1391. Unfortunately, the NOPHN had become increasingly dependent on outside contributions even though the membership had increased from 1,628 in 1917 to 3,360 by 1919. "Report of War Program Committee, January 22, 1918," NOPHN Collection, roll 25; Frances Payne Bolton, "The Work of the War Program Committee," *PHNQ* 10 (July 1918): 249–253; and Ella Crandall, "Organization Activities," *PHN* 14 (February 1920): 169.

123 "Annual Report of the Executive Secretary," NOPHN Collection, roll 11.

124 Fitzpatrick, *National Organization*, 64–68.

125 "Recommendations of the War Program Committee," [February 1918?], NOPHN Collection, roll 11; and "Report of the War Committee," January 22, 1918, NOPHN Collection, roll 22.

126 See note 122. At the time, 80 percent of the NOPHN members were nurses. Anne Stevens, "Activities of the NOPHN," *PHN* 3 (March 1922): 154; and Crandall, "Organization Activities," 169. Bolton discusses the wishes of the American Nurses Association (ANA) in "Recommendations of the War Program." Also see Fitzpatrick, *National Organization*, 24–25, for earlier concerns about lay membership.

127 Editorial, "The Chicago Meeting," *PHN* 11 (January 1919): 1–3. See also "Report of the Chicago Meeting," *PHN* 11 (January 1919): 152–161.

128 "Chicago Meeting," 2–3.

129 In fact, Gardner replaced Clements as director with Fox as assistant director. Gardner was to work part-time, acting as an advisor to Fox who was to become director at the end of the year. But when Gardner was sent to Europe by the Red Cross in September 1918, Fox became the director. Kernodle, *Red Cross Nurse*, 132, 134. Fox was a graduate of the University of Wisconsin and Johns Hopkins. She had worked on the staff of the Chicago VNA for four years; then at VNA of Dayton, Ohio; and later Washington, DC. In both Dayton and Washington, she was hired as superintendent with the express purpose of reorganization of the agency. Although Fox was seen as a friend of the NOPHN, her desire to avoid friction by assuming a "settled policy of soft pedal" made her a not very dependable or aggressive friend. Unfortunately, differences in background and personality between Fox and Noyes meant there was little harmony and therefore a lot of soft-pedaling. But as Crandall would later note, even if Noyes and Delano had been removed, "the ruthless arbitrariness governing the Red Cross would still be so entrenched as to limit their [Gardner/Fox] freedom of action." Ella Crandall to Mary Beard, February 19, 1919, Wald Collection, roll 31. See also Dock, *Red Cross*, 1274–1276; Fitzpatrick, *National Organization*, 81–82; and Kernodle, *Red Cross Nurse*, 244, 132.

130 "Chicago Meeting," 155.

131 Kernodle, *Red Cross Nurse*, 132.

132 Ibid.

133 The Red Cross even went so far as to, on three occasions, attempt to convince Kath-arine Olmstead, who ran the NOPHN Chicago office, to break her contract with the NOPHN to go with the Red Cross. Ella Crandall to Mary Beard, February 19, 1919, Wald Collection, roll 31.

134 Ibid.

135 Crandall is quoted in Brainard, *Evolution*, 359.

136 Bessie Amerman Haasis, "A Wartime Convention," *PHNQ* 10 (July 1918): 253–256.

137 George Rosen, "The Structure of American Medical Practice, 1875–1975," unpublished paper.

138 "Chicago Meeting," 152–161. For the effects of draft rejections on public opinion, see also IDNA of Boston, *Annual Report* (1917), 11; Frank Keefer, "Causes of Army Rejections: What Health Officers Can Do to Remedy Conditions," *AJPH* 10 (March 1920): 236–239; and "Physical Disqualifications as Shown by the Draft," *PHN* 11 (January 1919): 59–62. For the effect of the 1918 epidemic, see A. A. Hoehling, *The Great Epidemic* (Boston: Little, Brown, 1961). The Philadelphia Society cared for 4,050 patients during the epidemic between September 14 and November 2. Minutes of the Managers Meeting, VNS of Philadelphia, November 1918. IDNA staff realized during the epidemic that many people they cared for had never heard of their organization. But since they visited 40 percent (31,601) of the population during the epidemic, they assumed this situation had been radically improved. An additional outcome was a sustained increase in the number of volunteers. IDNA of Boston, *Annual Report* (1918), 13. The work of the Providence association during the epidemic is discussed in the DNA of Providence, *Annual Report* (1918), 17–19.

139 "Chicago Meeting," 156–157.

140 Fitzpatrick, *National Organization*, 75; and Hillard, "Report of the Rockefeller Conference."

141 VNS of Philadelphia, *Annual Report* (1918), 17.

142 Mary Roberts, "Current Events and Trends in Nursing," *AJN* 39 (January 1939): 2.

Chapter 5 — The Decline of Public Health Nursing

 1 George Vincent to Adelaide Nutting, December 4, 1918, Goldmark Folder, MAN Collection. Between 1917 and 1918, the foundation had been approached by a wide variety of individuals and organizations eager to obtain funds for projects they believed would improve public health nursing's situation. These included Nutting at Teachers College, Wald at Henry Street, the president of Vassar College, the president of Western Reserve, Miss Elizabeth Kemper-Adams of War Service Training for Women College Students, and Mrs. John Blodgett and Miss Gertrude Martin of the Association of Collegiate Alumnae. The fact that emerged from these various proposals was the lack of agreement among those most interested. The foundation's interest in public health nursing education evolved as a result of their wartime efforts to train visiteuses d'hygiene and their need for a similar worker in their broader public health work. History 900–902, "Source Material," vol. 8, RF Archives, pp. 2089–2090; and Resume of Rockefeller Foundation public health nursing and nursing education activities, RF Archives, 906, p. 1. For correspondence and minutes of the committee, see Goldmark folder, MAN Collection. For summary of the conference, see RF Archives, 200c, box 121.

2 Mrs. William Putnam to George Vincent, January 9, 1919; and James Miller to George Vincent, January 3, 1919. Emerson's idea to use health visitors in his health department originated with Miller. 200c, box 121, Rockefeller Foundation.

3 Adelaide Nutting to George Vincent. Winslow, in his usual supportive manner, replied to Nutting that this was indeed a great opportunity and congratulated her on being "very far sighted to seize upon it so promptly and effectively as you did." C.-E. A. Winslow to Adelaide Nutting, March 7, 1919, Winslow Collection, 21:1534.

4 Goldmark was the author of a well-received study of fatigue in women sponsored by the Russell Sage Foundation and other studies of social problems. Anne Strong—director of the postgraduate course at Simmons College, a classmate of Goldmark at Bryn Mawr who had been on the staff at Henry Street, and a teacher at Teachers College—was hired to assist Goldmark. Winslow, Beard, and Nutting served as the executive committee for the study. Nothing was left to chance. C.-E. A. Winslow to Embree, November 5, 1919, and C.-E. A; Winslow to Adelaide Nutting, June 27, 1919, MAN Collection; and Committee on Public Health Education Report of the Secretary, December 6, 11, 1920, MAN Collection. By February of 1920, Goldmark had reached some tentative conclusions, all acceptable to nursing. The same month, the foundation sponsored a second conference, and as a result, the study was extended to include all nursing education. Committee on the Study of Public Health Nursing Education, Report of the Secretary, February 11, 1920, Rockefeller Foundation History 900–902; 2098–2104.

5 See, for example, the Instructive District Nursing Association (IDNA) of Boston, *Annual Report* (1919), 12–13. Beard was finally able to resign as president of the National Organization for Public Health Nursing (NOPHN) the summer of 1919 and returned home from Washington, DC, ready at last to fully implement the plans for the IDNA she had initiated in 1915. Gardner returned the same year from Italy and service with the American Red Cross.

6 Ibid.; and see discussion, Minutes of the Board of Managers, Visiting Nurse Society (VNS) of Philadelphia, May 28, 1920.

7 Isabel Lowman, "Social Responsibility for Adequate Nurse's Salaries," *PHN* 12 (May 1920): 406–414.

8 Ibid.

9 The meeting was called at the suggestion of the IDNA of Boston. Representatives from the American Red Cross, the National Tuberculosis Association, the NOPHN, the Federal Children's Bureau, the Metropolitan Life Insurance Company (MLI), and visiting nurse associations (VNAs) from nine cities attended. The VNAs were from Providence, Philadelphia, Detroit, Henry Street Settlement House, Chicago, Baltimore, Cleveland, Brooklyn, and Boston. See IDNA of Boston, *Annual Report* (1919), 13; and "Summary" Report of NOPHN meeting, January 14, 1920, Winslow Collection, 87:1416. Philadelphia's calculations of average expenses included yearly work expenses such as uniforms, collars, shoes, gloves, and so on; personal expenses—hats, dresses, petticoats, corsets, nightgowns, vacations, and doctor's bills; and monthly expenses—food, rent, laundry, alumni expenses, magazines, and recreation. The total of $1,080 per year ironically matched exactly the annual salary the VNS paid its staff. VNS of Philadelphia, "Average Expenses of Staff 1919."

10 Mrs. Lowman was the chosen preacher, and her audience was the "nonprofessional members section"—that is, board members. She chose to discuss salaries in terms of a social responsibility of boards, assuring her audiences that if they followed the example of the larger organizations, they too could make significant contributions

to the extension of the work of the public health nurse. Her paper was later published in the *PHN*. Lowman, "Social Responsibility." For documentation of the increase in salary, see "Memorandum re Staff Salaries in Other Places," Minutes of the Nurse Committee, VNS of Philadelphia, May 3, 1922. For results of the salary survey, which included thirty cities, see "The Salary Question," *PHN* 15 (September 1923): 481–483. Increasing salaries certainly did have an impact on the larger associations. For example, while IDNA's staff increased by 25 percent, its budgets increased 43 percent from $151,000 in 1919 to $216,000 in 1920. In 1919, patient fees and MLI contributed 23 percent of the IDNA's income, and by 1920, this had increased to 29 percent. Boston ended the year with an $8,100 deficit. IDNA of Boston, *Annual Report* (1919), 35–40; and (1920), 31–32. See also Mary Beard, "A Review," IDNA, September 1921, 3. The VNS of Philadelphia added twenty-three nurses (35 percent increase) to their staff and $25,000 to their budget between 1920 and 1921. VNS of Philadelphia, *Annual Report* (1920), 8; and (1921), 11. The Providence District Nursing Association (DNA) had a comparable 37 percent increase in staff but a smaller increase in budget, no doubt due at least in part to their low salary scale. DNA of Providence, *Annual Report* (1920), 21; and (1922), 21. Of all the organizations surveyed for the January 1920 meeting, Providence paid the lowest salaries. See "Nurse Committee Notes," VNS of Philadelphia, 1919.

11 In Philadelphia, for example, the nurses were especially concerned about low salary, claiming they were paid a subsistence wage. In March 1925, Tucker told the board that it was simply a question of policy and that the nurses must be paid a higher salary, even if it meant the number of staff and therefore the volume of work had to be reduced. Not surprisingly, the board voted to increase salaries. Tucker claimed that except for Baltimore and Washington, DC, Philadelphia nurses were the lowest paid of any large organization. In actuality, of all organizations, they paid the twelfth highest salary. Board of Managers Meeting, VNS of Philadelphia, January 16, 1925; March 6, 1923; and March 13, 1925. Tucker believed the staff needed to increase by ten to twenty nurses. In one week in 1924, they had to turn away 125 cases, and since priority was given to the acutely ill, they usually refused normal maternity patients and the chronically ill. Board of Managers, VNS of Philadelphia, January 13, 20, 24, 25, 1922; February 24, 1922; April 28, 1922; and January 23, 1925. In Boston, Beard used a similar approach to raise the nurses' salary. Had the board failed to raise the money, she planned to decrease the number of staff by enough to pay those remaining a "living wage." Nurse Committee, November 12, 1923; and the Board of Managers, December 21, 1923, IDNA of Boston. The salary paid in twelve larger VNAs in 1924 and the 1924 analysis of staff living expenses for Philadelphia can be found in the Nurse Committee Report, 1924, VNS of Philadelphia.

12 Louis Dublin, "Records of Public Health Nursing," Lecture V, *PHN* 14 (January 1922): 17–24. Dublin's claims that this was a precarious situation are substantiated by the annual reports of the IDNA, VNS of Philadelphia, Henry Street Settlement, and DNA of Providence.

13 Ibid. The only new program introduced by the VNAs during this period was in mental hygiene, which was, in comparison to their last projects, very limited. See, for example, Gardner, *Public Health Nursing*, 343–359. This was the general agreement reached by those attending the general session of the NOPHN that followed a session titled, "Meeting the Demands for Community Health Work." They are summarized in Mary Gardner, "What Are Voluntary Organizations Going to Do about

Meeting Their Demands with the Funds Available?," *PHN* 16 (September 1924): 457–458.

14   "Appraisal of Insurance Visiting Nurse Work," unpublished study conducted by the MLI in 1923 as a supplement to the visiting nurse study conducted by the NOPHN, MLI Archives, New York, p. 22.

15   IDNA of Boston, *Annual Report* (1919), 35–44; (1920), 31; (1922), 213–233; (1923), 12; and (1924), 8–10.

16   Gardner discusses these traditional methods in "What Are Voluntary Organizations Going to Do?," 458.

17   Executive Committee Meeting, IDNA of Boston, January 20, 1920.

18   Ibid., March 4, 10, 31, 1920.

19   Executive Committee Meeting IDNA of Boston, March 12, 1920; July 30, 1920; and December 10, 1920. These fundraising methods were apparently considered successful enough for Miss Gertrude Peabody, vice president of the board of managers, to publish. Gertrude Peabody, "Opportunities and Responsibilities for Lay Persons in Public Health Nursing Work," *PHN* 16 (May 1924): 229–234.

20   A male executive committee of nine members was appointed in 1920. The result was not as successful as anticipated, since men were not willing to devote as much time as the ladies. Eventually, the ladies began to complain that since the men had been added, the meetings were shorter and less time was taken to discuss "all phases of the work." Nurse Committee Meetings IDNA of Boston, February 29, 1925. Local committees were mildly successful in fundraising. The board also decided that the office work should be reorganized and in July 1920 asked the NOPHN to release Miss Hale, a member of their staff, for a month to conduct a study of their office situation. Her study was completed on December 1920 and recommended replacing the volunteer office staff with a paid staff. Nurse Committee Meetings IDNA of Boston, February 29, 1925.

21   Ibid. Minutes of the Executive Committee Meeting, IDNA of Boston, February 28, 1923. Beard was first asked to report to the board on ways to limit the work in January 1923. At that time, she told the board she found the idea very difficult because what they were suggesting would mean reduction first in health promotion activities, second in prevention of disease, and third in the care of the sick. She was able to convince the board to make one last effort to raise the money needed to continue their present activities. Beard discussed her report to the board with the supervisors at their regular meeting on January 2, 1923. Minutes of the Supervisors Meeting, IDNA, January 21, 1923. IDNA's financial difficulties had apparently been heightened when in October 1922, they merged with the Baby Hygiene Association to form the CHA. As a result, CHA took on all the child welfare work in the city, and their staff increased from 123 to 161 nurses. See CHA of Boston, *Annual Report* (1922); and Mary Beard, "The Community Health Association of Boston: An Outline of the Plan of Organization following Combining the Work of the Instructive District Nurse Association and the Baby Hygiene Association," *PHN* 15 (March 1923): 115–118. Minutes of the Supervisors Meeting, CHA, November 12, 1923.

22   At the April 1, 1924, supervisors meeting, the question of eliminating work in anticipation of staff reductions was first discussed. By the April 16, 1924, supervisors meeting, Beard's frustration was apparent when she described the staff's continued cooperation as "remarkable." They had been asked to endure a great deal. They were generalists who were asked to become specialists; having become specialists,

they were then asked to again become generalists. They were then asked to extend their work to the whole community and finally were told they had gone too far and must limit their work. For the sake of the staff, she hoped the board would stand by whatever plan they chose for at least a year. Ironically, it was not until September 1923 that Beard finally succeeded in implementing to her full satisfaction the plans she had initiated in 1915. See Minutes of the Executive Committee, CHA, September 19, 1923.

Thus they had only been in place for seven months when the board decided to limit the work.

23 Despite her frustration and disappointment, the cuts had to come from somewhere. In her opinion, they should come from either maternity, chronic, or child health work, not from services to the acutely ill or services that were growing and paying for themselves. The supervisors had already paid a great deal of attention to the chronic cases and had substantially cut the numbers of visits made. Since no one else would care for such chronic patients, it would be difficult to further curtail this service. As for child health, Beard had been negotiating for over a year with the mayor and the health department to obtain city money to continue this service. They had even discussed amalgamating both staffs into a single agency under the control of CHA. Unfortunately, the health department not only decided against this plan but also concluded that the only way the city could get money to take over child health work was if CHA publicly stated they could no longer support it and turned it over to the health department. In Beard's opinion, this was not a very desirable choice because the health department was not yet in a position to "keep up the standards of the work." For this reason, she very much regretted having to give to them any aspect of the work she helped develop. On May 23, 1924, the supervisors decided to try to limit their work with preschool children, and on July 1, 1924, they voted to discharge all prenatal patients except those with MLI coverage who planned to deliver in the hospital. Minutes of the Nurses Committee, April 14, 1924; and Minutes of the Supervisors, April 16, 1924. For negotiations with the health department, see Minutes of the Nurse Committee, June 27, 1923; August 6, 1923; September 6, 1923; September 8, 1923; November 12, 1923; and May 14, 1924. For Beard's views on the health department standards, see Mary Beard to David Edsal, January 10, 1921.

24 The immediate crisis was finally resolved in August when the health department took over all child health work making it possible to reduce the staff by fifty nurses. They ended the year, no doubt much wiser, with a deficit of $57,881. The $130,000 reductions in expenses were no longer necessary. Minutes of the Board of Directors Meeting, May 10, 1921; July 18, 1921; August 9, 1921; and October 10, 1924. CHA of Boston, *Annual Report* (1924), 3–8; and (1925), 16. Beard, who had been trying to resign since 1921, again submitted her resignation, as did the executive committee in August. Neither was accepted. Minutes of the Board, CHA of Boston, June 28, 1924; and August 26, 1924. Beard first tried to resign May 10, 1921. The board decided to ask Crandall, who by that time had left the NOPHN, to take her place, but she declined and suggested they contact Tucker of Philadelphia or Mary Laird of Rochester. When they both declined, the board decided that perhaps after a good vacation, Beard might reconsider and voted to leave her position open until January. Her next attempt was in June 1924 and then again in August 1924. The board convinced her to take her vacation and a two month leave of absence at half-salary. In October, she wrote the board asking for a six month leave of absence to do

a "piece of work" for the Rockefeller Foundation. Since she was unwilling to guarantee her return at that time, the board finally accepted her resignation. Although Beard was offered the directorship of Henry Street, she decided to work for the International Health Division of the Rockefeller Foundation on a study of maternity care. In 1925, at the completion of this study, she became a special assistant to the director of Studies Division, traveling extensively throughout Europe. In 1938, she became director of the Red Cross Nursing Service and retired in 1944. "Mary Beard Dies," 29.

25 The main focus of the June 1928 convention, which was held in Detroit, centered on the issue of community demand for expanded services and the related issue of increased funding. See, for example, "High Visibility in the Convention Program," *PHN* 16 (April 1924): 167–170. Many of the papers presented at the convention can be found in the September and October issues of the *PHN*. Of the 5,000 people attending the combined convention (NLNE, ANA, NOPHN), 957 were members of the NOPHN; 883 of these were nurses, and the remainder were lay members. This registration was double that of past years. "Activities of NOPHN," *PHN* 16 (September 1924): 363. Beginning with the June 1924 *PHN*, a new series was begun at the suggestion of "the director of one of the large visiting nurse services" to discuss just these sorts of problems and policies. This new department was designed to offer an opportunity "for the flappers" of public health nursing to display their latest and most extreme innovations in management of the public health visit and to explain the broad and lasting results achieved on a small investment; it also offered the conservative an equal opportunity to defend "her low heels, steady gait and reverence for tradition." Florence Patterson, "A New Department and a New Series," *PHN* 16 (June 1924): 273–274. Patterson became director of the CHA of Boston when Beard resigned in October 1924.

26 It should be noted that three papers of this title were given at the convention, but Norton's was the focus of the round table discussion chaired by Gardner. The other papers were much more general and addressed the issues of educating the public and community demand for care. On the basis of Gardner's report of the discussion, it seems reasonable to assume that Norton's paper most directly addressed the issues most critical to the participants. William Norton, "Meeting the Demands for Community Health Work," *PHN* 16 (September 1924): 490–493. The other papers by the same title were by Haven Emerson, *PHN* 16 (September 1924): 485–489; and Ella Crandall, *PHN* 16 (October 1924): 506–512. A similar paper was also presented by Mrs. William Lee, "Obligations of the Board to Educate the Community in the Matter of Public Health Nursing," *PHN* 16 (September 1924): 495–497. Norton's paper was still being quoted two years later. Dorothy Deming, "Business Methods in Visiting Nurse Associations," *PHN* 18 (September 1926): 490–493. For a summation of the round table discussion, see Gardner, "What Are Voluntary Organizations Going to Do?"

27 Norton, "Meeting the Demands."

28 See, for example, Eleanor Marsh, "Telling the Public about the Public Health Nurse," *PHN* 12 (March 1920): 218–222; Sherman Kingsley, "Principles and Methods of Money Raising," *PHN* 12 (June 1920): 511–519; Estelle Hunter, "The Essentials of Office Management," *PHN* 12 (May 1920): 397–405; Sophie Nelson, "The Question of Community Funds," *PHN* 16 (March 1924): 124–126; and Anna Behr, "Publicity, an Essential Part of the Public Health Nursing Program," *PHN* 16 (January 1924): 21–26.

29   This notion about Boston was reported in the Minutes of the Managers Meeting, VNS of Philadelphia, October 31, 1924. They concluded that the initiation of a community fund drive would be inevitable, noting CHA's $80,000 deficit as sufficient evidence.

       Philadelphia had by that time formed a Welfare Federation; and Philadelphia, in 1920, had 439 agencies doing some kind of "social work" with aggregate budgets of between $19–$20 million. Kingsley, "Principles and Methods," 512.

30   Gardner, "What Are Voluntary Organizations Going to Do?," 457.

31   Ibid., 458. In fact, the number of new public health nursing associations (PHNAs) opening each year had been declining since 1920, which was a peak year with the formation of 441 new associations; by 1921, this number had declined to 301, and in 1923, only 238 new associations opened. Louise Tattershall, "Census of Public Health Nursing in the United States," *PHN* 18 (May 1926): 264.

32   In his paper, Frankel suggested to his audience that standardized financial statements would allow VNAs to begin to make comparisons from year to year and between organizations, thus allowing them to evaluate their successes and failures. Lee Frankel, "Standardization of Financial Statements for Visiting Nurse Associations," *PHNQ* 8 (July 1916): 67–71.

33   Katharine Codman became chair of the committee in January 1917. Report of the Committee on Organization and Administration, December 31, 1917, NOPHN Collection, roll 25.

34   For a discussion of Dr. Codman and his end result activities, see Reverby, "Stealing the Golden Eggs," 156–171.

35   According to Mrs. Codman, her committee accomplished little the first year, their major achievement being a meeting on duties and opportunities for direction and a round table discussion on the treasurer's statements at the convention. In July, they had begun to examine the question of standardized treasurers' reports, using Philadelphia as a model. They were also interested in salaries and methods of estimating cost. By 1919, Codman wrote Crandall to apologize for the lack of work accomplished by her committee and to share her plans for a small study of seven to eight large organizations and four to five smaller ones in terms of types of services provided and cost per visit. Report of the Committee on Organization and Administration, June 1918 and March 5, 1919, NOPHN Collection, roll 25. As a result of the round table discussion, several board members learned that MLI was reimbursing them at different rates and in different ways. While some found this disturbing, Mrs. Codman found it less than shocking "because each individual had dealt with Dr. Frankel separately. I think he makes the best possible arrangements he can." All agreed that it was important that they begin to keep uniform accounts so that they could compare their expenses and find out "whether we were getting the right amount of service for the money we were spending." Report of the Committee on Organization and Administration, May 17, 1918, NOPHN Collection, roll 35.

36   Actually, the first study was of the VNA of Cleveland, which was included in Haven Emerson, *The Cleveland Hospital and Health Survey* (Cleveland: Cleveland Hospital Council, 1920). The results of this study and some of its costs were included in the Goldmark Report. Another even smaller study was conducted by Goodrich in 1921. This was an analysis of the cost per visit of the Henry Street VNA. Marguerite Wales mentions this VNA study in "Time and Cost Study Problems," *PHN* 20 (March 1928): 138. This was not her first such analysis. In 1891, Goodrich conducted probably the first nursing time study. This study is discussed

in Susan Reverby, "The Nursing Disorder: A Critical History of the Hospital-Nursing Relationship, 1860–1945" (PhD diss., Boston University, 1982). The first substantial analysis of public health nursing was Goldmark, *Nursing and Nursing Education.*

37 Goldmark, *Nursing and Nursing Education*, 7–30, 109; and Adelaide Nutting, "Thirty Years of Progress in Nursing," in *Proceedings of the Twenty-Ninth Annual Convention of the National League for Nursing Education* (Baltimore, Md.: Williams & Wilkins, 1923), 109–115. The same reviewer went on to comment that "many of us are very much heartened to be assured that we have not been on the wrong track these last ten years and that the conclusion reached by this impartial high tribunal are the same as those reached by the most far-seeing of our own profession of nursing." Hillard, "Discussion of the Report," 176. For the comments of other reviewers, see, for example, Rate Douglas, "A Report of the Committee on the Study of Nursing Education," *Pacific Coast Journal of Nursing* 18 (1922): 563–564; Mary Gardner, "Library Department Book Notes," *PHN* 15 (May 1923): 260–263; "Improving Schools of Nursing: The Winslow Report in Retrospect," *Trained Nurse and Hospital Review* 71 (July 1923): 49–51; Richard Beard, "The Report of the Rockefeller Foundation on Nursing Education: A Review and Critique," *AJN* 23 (February/March 1923): 358–365 and 460–466; and "Committee on Nursing Education Issues Notable Report," *Modern Hospital* 19 (August 1922): 95–101.

38 The final committee had nineteen members, five of whom were nurses. The remaining members were predominantly physicians plus a few social workers. For a list of committee members, see Goldmark, *Nursing and Nursing Education*, 30.

39 Anne Strong to C.-E. A. Winslow, September 23, 1922, Winslow Collection, 61:711.

40 Goldmark, *Nursing and Nursing Education*, 10–30, 53, 137–139, 146.

41 Ibid., 83–117, 146.

42 C.-E. A. Winslow to Herman Biggs, Winslow Collection, 61:711. Ibid., 43, 10–29.

43 For a summary of the significance of the committee's conclusions for public health nursing, see Mary Beard, "Discussion of the Rockefeller Report: Analysis of the Situation in the Public Health Field," in *Proceedings of the Twenty-Ninth Annual Convention*, 179–184. By 1924, there were only thirty agencies where voluntary and official agencies had formed a single, amalgamated program. From the data presented in the 1924 census, it is clear that beyond the few instances, it was very uncommon for nurses working in official agencies to provide bedside care. This was later documented in the 1931 NOPHN survey as well. See Tattershall, "Census of Public Health Nursing," 262, 265; and NOPHN, *Survey of Public Health Nursing.* Lack of any significant reform of nursing education was later documented by May Burgess, *Nurses, Patients, and Pocketbooks* (New York: Committee on the Grading of Nursing Schools, 1928). Visiting nursing never really embraced the idea of the attendant, even when the growing number of chronic patients forced the question by the late 1920s. By that time, there was an oversupply of public health nurses, and their salaries were so low that hiring attendants had become nearly as expensive as using nurses. For example, the IDNA of Boston first talked about hiring attendants to care for chronic patients in 1927 and by 1929 had a grand total of two on the staff. The attendants' work was supervised by the nurses and was found to be acceptable, and most supervisors felt they "could use a few attendants" in their district. See Minutes of the Nurse Committee, CHA of Boston, November 22, 1926; and Minutes of the Board of Managers, CHA of Boston, October 25, 1929; and November 20, 1929.

44　Metropolitan Life Insurance, *Report of the Committee to Study Visiting Nursing Instituted by the NOPHN at the Request of the Metropolitan Life Insurance Company* (New York: Metropolitan Life Insurance, 1924), 95. Frankel apparently tired of waiting for Mrs. Codman's committee to address the issues he had first raised in 1916 and decided to take matters into his own hands. See notes 33–35. The committee had failed to make progress, and the MLI's series of articles on recordkeeping had no significant impact. See, for example, Lois Dublin, "Records of Public Health Nursing and Their Service in Casework, Administration and Research," *PHN* 13 (June 1921): 285–292; and Lois Dublin, "Records of Public Health Nursing: Tabulation and Analysis of Nursing Records," *PHN* 13 (October 1921): 518–531. Finally, on December 23, 1921, he wrote the NOPHN, calling their attention, again, to the need for an impartial and unbiased study "of the work of visiting nurse associations, that examined both quality and quantity." *Committee to Study Visiting Nursing,* 12–13. Frankel's letter was discussed at the January meeting of the executive committee of the NOPHN, and his offer to pay for the study was accepted. Minutes of the Executive Committee Meeting of NOPHN, January 16–18, 1922, NOPHN Collection, roll 11. The final report was presented and approved at the 1924 NOPHN convention. See "Report of Round Table on Visiting Nursing Study," June 20, 1924, Winslow Collection, 87:1416.

45　Metropolitan Life Insurance, *Report of the Committee to Study.* The committee was provided a $15,000 budget. They attempted to get Josephine Goldmark to conduct the study, but she was not available. Minutes of the Executive Committee, NOPHN, February 12–16, 1922; and September 18–19, 1922, NOPHN Collection, roll 11.

46　Nine private, two public, and three semipublic organizations were surveyed: Philadelphia, Boston, Cleveland, Louisville, Denver, Portland, Indianapolis, Omaha, Oklahoma City, New Orleans, Los Angeles, Rochester, York, and either Manhattan/ Bronx or Brooklyn. "Appraisal of Insurance," p. 22; and Minutes of the Executive Committee, NOPHN, September 18–19, 1922; and October 30–November 1, 1922, NOPHN Collection, roll 11. The committee's original title, Visiting Nurse Association Appraisal Study Committee, was, for some unstated reason, changed to the Committee to Study Visiting Nursing. The survey was conducted by a trained researcher, two nurses, and an accountant. One of the nurses was Janet Geister who had also been an investigator with the Goldmark Study and who was the field and later educational secretary of the NOPHN. Minutes of the Executive Committee, October 30–November 1, 1922, roll 11; and *Committee to Study Visiting Nursing,* 11–14, 93. Among other things, the study found that the average age of the staff was thirty-three, 72 percent were high school graduates, 10 percent had attended college, and only 25 percent had any advanced training in public health nursing. Only three of the fourteen agencies required experience in public health for employment. The average staff turnover was 36 percent, while in some agencies, it was as high as 80 percent. The range of length of employment for administrators was three to eight years and for nursing staff two to four years, while the average salary was $125/week. While 92 percent of the administrators belonged to the NOPHN, only 47 percent of the staff were members. Finally, the majority of care provided by the organizations surveyed was free. *Committee to Study Visiting Nursing,* 46–52, 70, 84–86, 94–95, 105–107.

47　Metropolitan Life Insurance. *Report of the Committee to Study,* 11, 76, 98–100, 105–108.

48　Ibid., 15–19.

49 "The Report on Visiting Nursing," *Nation's Health* (January 1925): 6. This review was written by Mrs. Susa Moore, associate editor of *Nation's Health*, and was a much diluted version of her views, the result of numerous letters between William Snow, chairman of the committee, and Moore. After a couple of letters, Snow started sending copies to the other committee members and eventually sought the advice of Winslow, who, at the time was the editor of *Nation's Health*. Winslow had reviewed and substantially changed Moore's piece before it was published. But he wrote in response to Snow's note that although his editing had made her report less unfavorable, "It seems to me in rereading this statement that I did not perhaps edit it sufficiently." Unable to account for the cause of her grievance, he concluded she was some kind of "grouch" and apologized for her rather curt and ungracious report. Although Winslow asked that Snow write an editorial, one never appeared. In her letters, she questioned MLI motives in funding the study, questioned the judgment and conclusions of the researcher, found its failure to correlate findings a disappointment, was left wondering where visiting nursing might fit into the health scheme, and in general found the study dull and hardly inspirational. In contrast, Winslow reassured Snow that he found the report a valuable and constructive contribution to a difficult subject. Susa Moore to William Snow, January 5, 1925; January 15, 1925; January 29, 1925; William Snow to Susa Moore, January 10, 1925; January 22, 1925; March 7, 1925; William Snow to C.-E. A. Winslow, March 7, 1925; and C.-E. A. Winslow to William Snow, March 16, 1925, Winslow Collection, 88:1423.

50 "Report of Round Table," p. 2. In fact, Frankel had been conducting his own study, and while publicly expressing his gratitude for the committee work, he was also suggesting the need for more study of the issues raised by his study. "Appraisal of Insurance." Gardner told the participants that she and her staff had reviewed the recommendations and found them "quite practicable." Tucker stated her organization had already tried them out and found them "workable." "Report of Round Table." Tucker had in fact gone much farther than the recommendations as a result of the study. She now required her staff to record their time spent in visits, transportation, office and records work, and so on, and each month, these data were posted so that each nurse could analyze her own "productivity." Minutes of the Board of Managers, VNS of Philadelphia, June 6, 1924.

51 Marguerite Wales, "The Value of Measuring Rods in a Visiting Nurse Service," *PHN* 19 (March 1927): 117–121; Wales, "Time and Cost," 138–140; Emma Winslow, "Service Norms and Their Variation," *PHN* 22 (February 1930): 68–73; and (March 1930): 151–152; Emma Winslow, "The Measurement of Nurse Power," PHN 19 (September 1927): 492–498; Emilie Sargent, "More about Measuring Rods," *PHN* 19 (May 1927): 231–233; Ira Hiscock, "The Value of Records and the Annual Report," *PHN* 19 (March 1927): 167–171; Emma Winslow, "Service Costs and Program Planning," *PHN* 20 (November 1928): 569–574; W. F. Walker, "The Appraisal of Nursing Service," *PHN* 20 (October 1928): 518–524; Emma Winslow, "More about the Measurement of Nurse Power," *PHN* 20 (February 1928): 63–68; and Burgess, *Nurses, Patients, and Pocketbooks*. Having completed its study, the Committee to Study Visiting Nursing broadened its focus, and in 1927, changed its title to Service Evaluating Committee. Minutes of the Executive Committee, NOPHN, April 27, 1927, roll 11. In October, they decided that they should again examine the issue of calculating the cost of a visit. With the experience of the past few years, agencies had found the recommended method of total cost / total visits both unfair and crude.

They were also eager to study the effect of educational health services in preventing acute illnesses among young insurance policyholders.

   They planned to ask the insurance companies to finance these studies. Minutes of the Service Evaluation Committee of NOPHN, October 5, 1927; and January 16, 1928, roll 14. Jane Allen, "Report of the Service Evaluation Committee," *PHN* 19 (December 1927): 622. After much discussion, the study had not begun in 1929. They had requested $12,000 for the study, but Frankel felt such an extensive study was unnecessary and convinced the committee to confine themselves to a mail questionnaire surveying only twenty-four agencies. Their ultimate goal was to determine cost/minute. The underlying issue was of course for them to find, from the perspective of the VNA, the most favorable method to calculate reimbursement for visits made to "insurance" patients. Minutes of the Service Evaluation Committee of NOPHN, October 8, 1930, roll 14. Finally, another major demonstration that supported the views of the visiting nurse leadership was conducted at the East Harlem Health Center. See East Harlem Nursing and Health Service, *The Cost of a Program of Health Activities with Special Emphasis on Public Health Nursing* (New York: East Harlem Nursing and Health Service, 1926); and East Harlem Nursing and Health Service, *Comparative Study.*

52 Gardner, "What Are Voluntary Organizations Going to Do?," 457.

53 For a discussion of these ideas, see Rosenberg, "Inward Vision and Outward Glance," 346–391; Vogel, "Transformation," 105–116; and Susan Reverby, "The Search for the Hospital Yardstick: Nursing and the Rationalization of Hospital Work," in *Health Care in America*, 206–225; and "Ernest Amory Codman."

54 Minutes of the Executive Committee, NOPHN, March 10–11, 1925, NOPHN Collection, roll 11; and "Report of Conference of Representative of Voluntary (Non-official, Non-governmental) Private Public Health Associations," May 7, 1925, Wald Collection, roll 31.

55 Ibid. Patterson reported on the meeting at Nurses Committee Meeting, May 11, 1925, CHA of Boston.

56 Gardner, *Public Health Nursing*, 53, 69–74. These views were proclaimed in an editorial. Isabel Lowman, "The Question of Bedside Care," *PHN* 15 (February 1923): 55–56, and also by Mabelle Welch (of the East Harlem Nursing and Health Demonstration) in "A Public Forum," *PHN* 17 (April 1925): 214–216. Visiting nurses were correct in their belief that unlike VNAs, voluntary hospitals did have a long history as the recipients of governmental funds for provision of curative services. See Rosemary Stevens, "A Poor Sort of Memory: Voluntary Hospitals and Government before the Depression," *Milbank Memorial Fund Quarterly: Health Care and Society* 60 (Fall 1982): 551–584.

57 "Amalgamating of Public Health Nursing Service," *PHN* 17 (June 1925): 285. The campaign was launched in the June 1925 issue of the *PHN* when a series of articles were begun that would demonstrate "the trend of public health nursing services, and the possibilities of either amalgamation or federation which have so far revealed themselves." Up to this time, the only outstanding example of amalgamation was in Dayton, Ohio. This organization was created in 1914 by Fox, who, at the time was the superintendent of the Dayton VNA. See, for example, "The Coordination of Public and Private Agencies in the Conduct of a Completely Generalized Public Health Nursing Service," *AJPH* 12 (November 1922): 922–924. When Beard tried to get the city to merge all child health services within the CHA, she modeled her plan after Dayton. See note 21.

58 Ibid. This organizational solution was supported by the Goldmark Report, the East Harlem Study, and the Report of the Committee on Municipal Health Department Practices. The largest and most comprehensive was the East Harlem Study of generalized versus specialized nursing services that demonstrated beyond all doubt both the qualitative and quantitative superiority of a generalized program of care that combined curative and preventive services. The East Harlem Service was initiated in December 1922. See Goldmark, *Nursing and Nursing Education*, 8–10; and "Report of the Committee on Municipal Health Department Practice of the APHA in Cooperation with the United States Public Health Service," *Public Health Bulletin* 136 (July 1923): 154–156, 160–161. For examples of the articles and discussion of amalgamated nursing services, see Louise Orr, "How Evansville, Indiana Federated Its Nursing Services," *PHN* 17 (June 1925): 300–302; Elizabeth Holt, "Reorganization of Public Health Nursing in Dayton, Ohio," *PHN* 17 (October 1925): 520–522; Elizabeth Yost, "Reorganization of Public Health Nursing," *PHN* 17 (December 1925): 610–611; Mabelle Welch, "The Case for Generalization," *PHN* 18 (January 1926): 15–16; Jane Tuttle, "Coordination of Public Health Nursing Service in Columbus, Ohio," *PHN* 18 (September 1926): 509–510; Ellie Nelson, "Reorganization of Public Health Nursing Service, Charleston, S.C.," *PHN* 18 (June 1926): 359–364; Marguerite Clancy, "Reorganization of the Charleston, West Virginia Public Health Nursing Service," *PHN* 18 (February 1926): 80–82; Bettie McDonald, "Reorganization of Public Health Nursing Services of Louisville, Kentucky," *PHN* 18 (October 1926): 561–563; Netta Ford, "A Centralized Public Health Nursing Service, York, Pennsylvania," *PHN* 19 (February 1927): 89–91; Hulda Cron, "Federation of Nursing Services, Evansville and Vanderburgh County, Indiana," *PHN* 20 (April 1928): 193–195; and Helen Bond, "The Savannah Health Center," *PHN* 21 (November 1929): 593–596.

59 See, for example, Merrill Champion, "Again, What of the Public Health Nurse?," *PHN* 14 (February 1922): 67–69; "A Public Forum," *PHN* 17 (December 1925): 656; and Duffy, "American Medical Profession," 1–22.

60 Louise Tattershall, "Census of Public Health Nursing in the United States, 1931," *PHN* 24 (April 1932): 206.

61 It was their last study of combined agencies because after 1952, the NOPHN no longer existed. For a discussion of the NOPHN's final efforts in support of this idea, see Fitzpatrick, *National Organization*, 183–184. Their final study was conducted by the Committee on Nursing Administration and was entitled "The Project for the Study of Administration of Nursing Services in Combination Public Health Agencies," 1949, NOPHN Collection, roll 24. See also Dorothy Rusby, *A Study of Combination Services in Public Health Nursing* (New York: NOPHN, 1950).

62 Mary Gardner, "Modern Problems in the Public Health Nursing Field," *PHN* 21 (August 1929): 413–416; Frances Bolton, "A Cleveland Opinion of the Community Chest Idea," *PHN* 14 (December 1922): 610–614; Nelson, "Community Funds," 124–126; Gertrude Hussey, "What of the Community Chest?," *PHN* 20 (June 1928): 291–293; and Gardner, *Public Health Nursing*, 442–451.

63 See note 51. The visiting nurse study produced a great deal of interest on the part of those associations who participated in the study. As a result, they became much more interested in productivity, staff efficiency, and cost/service. For example, see Minutes of the Board of Managers, VNA of Philadelphia, June 6, 1924; DNA of Providence, *Annual Report* (1925); Minutes of the Nurse Committee, VNS of Philadelphia, November 11, 1928; Minutes of the Supervisors Meeting, CHA of Boston,

July 10, 1925; Deming, "Business Methods," *PHN* 18 (September 1926): 490–493; Wales, "Value of Measuring Rods," 118; Winslow, "Service Costs"; and Mrs. Richard Noye, "Financial Problems," *PHN* 19 (June 1927): 318–320.

64 Charging for care was not a new concept for most VNAs; it had just simply taken on a new level of significance. See chapter 3. Deming, "Business Methods"; and Elizabeth Fox, "The Economics of Nursing," *AJN* 29 (September 1929): 1037–1044. An alternative solution was attempted by the Manhattan Health Society. Their prepaid generalized nursing service lasted from 1922 to 1925. See Olive Husk, "The Manhattan Health Society," *PHN* 16 (January 1924): 27–32; and Olive Husk, "A Pioneer Self-Support Health Service," *PHN* 17 (April 1925): 184.

65 Hourly nursing was seen as the salvation of not only the visiting nurse but the private-duty nurse as well. The issue was not whether to pursue this solution for both groups of nurses but rather whether it should be organized by the VNAs or the private-duty registry. C.-E. A. Winslow, "The Nursing Problem," *New England Journal of Medicine* 200 (February 1929): 268; Michael Davis, "The Meaning of the Hourly Nursing Experiment in Chicago," *AJN* 33 (February 1933): 111–112; and Miriam Ames, "Hourly Nursing: Report of an Eighteen Month Experiment," *AJN* 33 (February 1933): 113–123. For an excellent discussion of the problems of private-duty nurses, see Susan Reverby, "Something besides Waiting: The Politics of Private Duty Nursing Reform in the Depression," in *Nursing History*, 133–156. See also Janet Geister, "Hearsay and Facts in Private Duty," *AJN* 26 (July 1926): 515–528.

For a description of hourly nursing from the perspective of the private-duty nurse, see Alma Wrigles, "The Hourly Nurse and Her Place," *AJN* 16 (April 1916): 874–881. In a comment at the end of this paper, Lent suggests that "rightly part of [hourly work] belongs to the VNA." See also Burgess, *Nurses, Patients, and Pocketbooks*, 349–353. While VNAs were opening hourly services, so were many registries. For example, in 1926, the Committee on Hourly Nursing decided to initiate an hourly service through a central registry. Minutes of the Nurse Committee, CHA of Boston, June 8, 1926. In Philadelphia, it was not until 1930 that the Central Nurses Registry decided to consider offering an hourly service. In February, they contacted the VNS to inquire if this would be encroaching upon their work. Minutes of the Nurse Committee, VNS of Philadelphia, February 21, 1930.

66 Ames, "Hourly Nursing"; and Davis, "Hourly Nursing Experiment."

67 Florence Patterson to C.-E. A. Winslow, November 11, 1926; and November 18, 1926, Winslow Collection, 34:55.

68 Ibid. Dorothy Deming, "One Way Out: An Answer to Some Problems of Private Duty Nursing." May Ayres Burgess, director of the committee on the Grading of Nursing Schools, sent a copy of the Deming article, which appeared in the June 1926 issue of the survey, to the members of her committee on July 12, 1926, MAN Collection. According to Gardner, unlike the poor, hourly patients had not yet learned to accept an "instructive service" without protest. Gardner, *Public Health Nursing*, 429. In an article describing their hourly service, the VNS of Philadelphia claimed the service was regarded as an "essential rounding out of the community health program." The nurses claimed they received a warm response from their hourly patients who were eager to follow their every instruction. The article fails to note that as late as 1927, most hourly visits were made to members of the VNS board. "Hourly Nursing Service," *PHN* 20 (March 1928): 126–128. Philadelphia VNA hourly service clientele were discussed at the May 23, 1927, executive meeting of the CHA of Boston.

69 It was generally agreed that chronic patients were those most often requesting hourly services; they were the patients who had the greatest difficulty obtaining institutionally based care. See, for example, Harriet Leek, "The Hartford Hourly Nursing Service," *PHN* 20 (May 1928): 238–240. See also the NOPHN's survey of the fifty-four organizations reportedly offering hourly services. Louise Tattershall, "Hourly Nursing in Public Health Nursing Associations," *PHN* 19 (August 1927): 397–402.

70 Ibid. Patterson to Winslow, November 11 and 18, 1926; Minutes of the Nurse Committee, CHA of Boston, May 27, 1930; and Minutes of the Board of Managers, CHA of Boston, May 28, 1928. For example, Patterson and her staff felt that the demand for hourly nursing should come from the community—from people interested in securing superior nursing services at a lower rate possible than with the full-time private-duty nurse. They were apparently content to wait for the community to eventually come to this realization and demand the service. Minutes of the Nurse Committee, CHA of Boston, May 28, 1928.

71 For the details of these activities, see Reverby, "Private Duty Nursing." The committee was appointed in 1928, but when by January 1930 it decided to focus on hourly nursing, the NOPHN decided to reconsider its representatives, making new appointments in light of this special emphasis. The NOPHN described the ANA as "much concerned by this hourly nursing service as it relates to registrars" and intended to actively protect the interests of VNAs. The committee gave their final report to Mary Roberts to be published in the *AJN*, but she was not interested, because she thought the information in the report would be of little assistance to her readers who saw in hourly nursing a way out of unemployment. The committee conducted a survey of hourly nursing in 1931 and 1932, talked about writing a manual on hourly nursing for communities considering establishing such a service, and published some tentative standards. Minutes of the Executive Committee Meeting of NOPHN, January 1930, NOPHN Collection, roll 11; Minutes of the Subcommittee on Hourly Appointment Service of the Committee on Distribution of Nursing Services, September 17, 1932; June 11, 1933; and January 20, 1934, NOPHN Collection, roll 26; and "The Hourly Appointment Nursing Service: Some Tentative Standards Prepared by the Joint Committee on Distribution of Nursing Service," *AJN* 31 (May 1931): 567–569.

72 The strongest public criticism came from Davis, but the MLI's unpublished "Appraisal of Insurance" drew similar conclusions about the VNA's missed opportunities.

73 Michael Davis, "Nursing Service Measured by Social Needs," *AJN* 39 (January 1939): 38–39. The results of the 1930 Rosenwald study can be found in Ames, "Hourly Nursing."

74 The 1927 study of the fifty-four organizations offering services concluded that although a need for hourly nursing existed, in those organizations where it was available, it only accounted for a small part (1–3 percent) of the work. Requests for service tended to come from patients rather than physicians, and the majority of patients requesting hourly services were chronically ill. Tattershall, "Hourly Nursing." This 1931 survey concluded that hourly nursing service as it was then conducted was not a success: it lacked funds for publicity, was without a clearly defined organizational plan, and was not recognized by the nursing staff as an enlarged opportunity for service. Minutes of the Subcommittee on Hourly Appointment Service of the Committee on Distribution of Nursing Services, September 17, 1932, NOPHN Collection, roll 26.

75 The Committee on Community Nursing was formed in 1934 but failed to do little more than what Susan Reverby called "fact finding and standard making." By the time Gardner wrote about the committee in 1936, it had a full-time secretary but had not, as yet, become active. Its purpose was to assist communities "upon their request" through consultation and advice, in meeting the need for a planned related and complete nursing service. See Reverby, "Private Duty Nursing"; and Gardner's chapter, "Bedside Care for the Patient of Moderate Means," in *Public Health Nursing*, 428–435.

76 By the mid-1920s, the John Hancock Mutual Life Insurance Company began to write industrial policies that included the services of visiting nurses. This helped to increase the income received by VNAs from the insurance companies. For exact figures, see financial statements included in the annual reports of most VNAs. For rather scattered overview of VNA sources of income for 1923 and 1924, see "Policies and Problems of PHN Services," *PHN* 17 (September/October 1925): 483–487 and 534–536. The 1927 average of earned income was 35 percent. "Earned Income of 29 Public Health Nursing Associations," *PHN* 21 (April 1929): 216.

77 Unlike the VNAs, who received essentially no public money, 18 percent of voluntary hospital income came from tax funds. See Stevens, "Poor Sort of Memory."

78 The decline was no doubt triggered by the depression and the resultant cancelation of policies but was continued by a growing dependence upon the hospital as the locus of medical care. In 1930, MLI paid for 5 million nursing visits at a cost of about $4.5 million, by the late 1940s, they paid for 1.5 million visits at a cost of nearly $4 million. At the same time, only 1 percent of MLI policyholders made use of the service. While by the time the MLI service was discontinued, the VNAs were already accustomed to obtaining a smaller percentage of the budget from MLI, it did have its impact. In Philadelphia, for example, it meant a 23 percent reduction. John Hancock terminated its nursing service the same year. See for a discussion of the changes in MLI service and an explanation of its termination, the last issue of *The Quarterly Bulletin for Metropolitan Nurses*, 15 (November 1951) in which the MLI both "bids adieu" and declares its "mission accomplished." See also "1909–1952 the Metropolitan Nursing Service Termination Announcement," MLI Archives; Alma Haupt, "Forty Years of Teamwork in Public Health Nursing," *AJN* 53 (January 1953): 81–84; and "A Report of a Study of the Effect of the Termination of Metropolitan Nursing Contracts," *PHN* 43 (May 1951): 285–292.

79 By the late 1920s, directors of some of the larger VNAs were finally ready to admit that "maybe" with the growing tendency toward hospitalization, visiting nurses would eventually be caring for fewer patients in their homes. Perhaps, suggested Tucker, the future development of visiting nursing would be more in the direction of quality and content than in quantity. VNA of Philadelphia, *Annual Report* (1928), 9. As early as 1928, she talked with Frankel of MLI inquiring if he knew of some other organization in the community doing their work that might account for the decrease in their service. They apparently concluded that at least some of their decline could be attributed to the hospitals and health centers. Minutes of the Board of Directors Meeting, VNS of Philadelphia, December 14, 1928. Some VNAs cautiously established referral systems with hospitals, correctly anticipating that these institutions would be most eager to pass on to them those patients unable to pay for their care. While most looked wherever they could for funds or ways to become more self-supporting, little seemed to change. See, for example, Minutes of the Nurse Committee, CHA of Boston, October 25, 1929; April 8, 1929; April, 22, 1929; and May 27, 1930.

80 For a further discussion of these changes, see Monroe Lerner and Odin Anderson, *Health Progress in the United States: 1900–1960* (Chicago: University of Chicago Press, 1963); and Condran and Cheney, "Mortality Trends."

81 Rosen, "First Neighborhood Health Center," 1620–1635. By the mid-1920s, the majority of VNA patients were native born and white. In 1927, for example, 44 percent of Philadelphia's VNA patients were native born / white, 23 percent were colored, and 32 percent foreign-born. VNS of Philadelphia, *Annual Report* (1927), 12. The new source of concern was the "colored situation" precipitated by massive migration from the South. This proved to be a greater problem for Philadelphia than Boston. Although the number of "colored cases" had been increasing since 1923, by 1929, work in colored districts had fallen off so much that they had to let go one (of their two) colored nurses, since "experience had proven that white families did not wish to employ a colored nurse." Minutes of the Nurse Committee, CHA of Boston, March 26, 1923; and March 11, 1929. In contrast, by 1927, Philadelphia's VNS was doing 24 percent of its work with colored patients, a dramatic increase from 17 percent in 1917. During that same period, it was claimed that Philadelphia's colored population had increased by 100 percent. Minutes of the Board of Managers, VNS of Philadelphia, February 25, 1927; and March 4, 1927. The approach of the VNS to its growing colored caseload was not unlike their turn-of-the-century view of immigrant families. In the 1922 annual report, the VNS of Philadelphia concluded that the "tremendous increase" in Negro population had created a comparable increase in "health problems for the city as a whole." "Surely there [was] no sounder and surer way," they suggested, "of helping these and other strangers within our gates to assimilate our standards and customs than through a health teacher in the home who shows through demonstration as well as precept how health can be made possible." VNS of Philadelphia, *Annual Report* (1922), 12.

82 For a discussion of the growth of the hospital, see Vogel, "Transformation," and "Hospital Services in the United States," *JAMA* 100 (March 1933): 887.

83 Katharine Tucker, "The Place and Value of Visiting Nursing in Community Health Work," *PHN* 14 (October 1922): 506. Tucker's agency, the VNS of Philadelphia, is an example of what happened to many associations. While in 1927 they made 270,000 visits to 33,000 patients, by 1958, this number had decreased to 141,000 visits to 12,000 patients. In the meantime, their annual budget increased from $252,000 to $583,000. In 1956, the VNA had a $24,000 deficit: 53 percent of the care given was free, while 18 percent was paid for by the patients, and 46 percent of their expenses were paid by the community chest. See VNS of Philadelphia, *Annual Report* (1922 and 1958).

84 Kernodle, *Red Cross Nurse in Action*, 239–258; Mary Gardner, "Under the American Red Cross," *PHN* 20 (November 1928): 597–599; Elizabeth Fox, "The Development of the Red Cross Bureau of Public Health Nursing," *PHN* 12 (February 1920): 175–181; and "The Correlation of National Social Agencies," *PHN* 13 (April 1921): 179.

85 According to the *Annual Report: Bureau of Public Health Nursing* for 1920–1921, Red Cross nurses could be found in the high Sierras, among Indian tepees, in the Appalachians, on islands off the New England coast, on the plains of Montana, and along the Mexican border. Several of their more spectacular adventures can be found in Dock, *Red Cross*, 1337–1351.

86 Fox, "Development"; Dock, *Red Cross*, 1286; and Kernodle, *Red Cross Nurse*, 251, 260–261.

87 Kernodle, *Red Cross Nurse*, 240, 261–262, 257.

88 Noyes was president of the ANA from 1918 to 1922, and Fox was president of the NOPHN from 1921 to 1926. Kernodle, *Red Cross Nurse*, 245–246. Dock, *Red Cross*, 1332–1333. Interestingly, when they published articles about the Red Cross, Fox's appeared in the *PHN*, while Noyes's were in the *AJN*. Noyes had been made director of the nursing division after the death of Delano.

89 Money was given to the programs at George Peabody College, Richmond School of Social Work, the Pennsylvania School for Social Service, and Simmons College. By the time the program ended in 1929, 730 scholarships and 446 loans had been given. Kernodle, *Red Cross Nurse*, 267–270; and Dock, *Red Cross*, 1286.

90 Dock, *Red Cross*. Kernodle, *Red Cross Nurse*, 262–263, 271–276, 240, 291–293. The agreements can be found in Dock, *Red Cross*, 1326–1331; "An Agreement between Three National Organizations," *PHN* 12 (February 1920): 162–163; and "The Relationship," *PHN* 13 (January 1921): 67–68. Ironically, one of the NOPHN assigned functions was to assist in organization and improvement of postgraduate courses, but in 1921, the Red Cross, according to Kernodle out of self-interest, gave money to the NOPHN Educational Committee to prevent its discontinuance because of a lack of funds. Kernodle, *Red Cross Nurse*, 253–254.

91 Ibid. Apparently, Farrand's and Fox's views differed from those of the district directors who resented the dictates that came from Washington, DC, to local chapters and who found the "autocratic ruling of the Red Cross so necessary in war" now unnecessary. "Report of the Western Office," May 1919, NOPHN Collection, roll 27. For an example of the variety of letters written by the Red Cross in its efforts to assure other organizations that it did not "contemplate the invasion of territory where other organizations are engaged in work of this character," see Rupert Blue (surgeon general public health service) to Mrs. Ira Perkins, chief, Child Conservation Section, Council of National Defense, Washington, April 3, 1919, National Archives, Public Health Service, General file 1897–1923:3815, box 372.

92 Boardman presented her views in a speech at the Red Cross National Convention of Chapter Delegates in October 1922. Kernodle, *Red Cross Nurse*, 240, 276–278, 285. According to Kernodle, Boardman had never before been such a "strict constructionist" of the Red Cross charter and hypothesized that Boardman would have felt less strongly if the Red Cross's expanding had not also included social work, a profession for which she felt a strong distaste.

93 As a result of Boardman's speech, the "Central Committee" met on December 13, 1922, and reaffirmed its commitment to their PHN programs. Boardman, adamant in her disapproval, turned her forces on organizing volunteer services. Kernodle, *Red Cross Nurse*, 277–278.

94 Ibid., 270, 263.

95 Ibid., 267–268, 272.

96 The study was conducted by Virginia Gibbs, began in the summer of 1921, and was published in September 1922. Dock, *Red Cross*, 1335. The findings are summarized in Elizabeth Fox, "Ratings of Red Cross Public Health Nurses and Their Interpretation," *PHN* 14 (September 1922): 270–272. By 1925, money for scholarships had been reduced to $1,500 a year and for loans to $3,000 per year. Kernodle, *Red Cross Nurse*, 269.

97 Kernodle, *Red Cross Nurse*, 283; Dock, *Red Cross*, 1332–1333; Elizabeth Fox, "Remodeling the Red Cross," *PHN* 13 (May 1921): 263–266; and Clara Noyes, "American Red Cross Reorganization," *AJN* 25 (March 1925): 224–225.

98   Kernodle, *Red Cross Nurse*, 257.

99   Ibid., 263, 282. Apparently, Fox wrote a series of articles for the Red Cross Courier in which she described what she had learned during those years in an effort to plan for future development. They were compiled and published in a pamphlet called *What the Future Holds for Public Health Nursing under the Red Cross* in 1928 and summarized in Gardner, "American Red Cross," 597–599.

100   Katharine Tucker, "Report of the General Director, Biennial Period 1928–1930," *PHN* 22 (July 1930): 346.

101   Tucker's paper borrowed heavily from one written by Ella Crandall, "NOPHN, What It Is and What It Does," NOPHN Collection, roll 27. Katharine Tucker, "Presidential Address to the National Organization for Public Health Nursing," *PHN* 12 (June 1920): 457–461. Similar views are found in editorials in *PHN*—for example, 12 (September 1920): 719–721; and 12 (August 1920): 651–654.

102   Tucker, "Presidential Address," 461.

103   Budgets between 1916 and 1919 are reviewed in "Statement from the NOPHN," Winslow Collection. The advisory committee voted to increase the budget from $74,000 to $174,000. Minutes of the Advisory Committee, November 15, 1919, NOPHN Collection, roll 28.

104   Foley expressed her views on these plans in a letter to Winslow. Edna Foley to C.-E. A. Winslow, December 23, 1920, Winslow Collection, 87:1391. Apparently, Wald and Nutting shared her views. Wald wrote to her that she thought the time had come to take stock of what work they could adequately perform now and do no more than that. She likewise did not approve of securing "big sums" from a few people. Lillian Wald to Edna Foley, November 15, 1920.

105   Edna Foley to Lillian Wald, November 19, 1920; and Edna Foley to Lillian Wald, December 29, 1920, Wald Collection.

106   Ibid. Foley described her relationship with Crandall as having not been one "of friendly and sympathetic intercourse."

107   The NOPHN did not accept her resignation until May. A few years later, she left nursing altogether. Her exit apparently left everyone surprised and some, like Wald, angry. Crandall was apparently reacting to the expanded responsibilities given to nonnurse members on the board of directors. "Radical Revision of By Laws," Annual Report of Executive Secretary, 1919, NOPHN Collection, roll 25. Crandall describes Wald's reaction in Eleanor Mumford, "Transcript of Field Interview with Ella Crandall," January 19, 1937, Gardner Papers, folder 45; and Fitzpatrick, *National Organization*, 92. They asked Beard to take the job, but she declined and in 1921 also resigned from the board because she "wished to be completely detached from professional responsibility." Eventually, Crandall was replaced by Patterson, who, in 1922, resigned to go to Boston to replace Beard at the IDNA. Edna Foley to Lillian Wald, September 26, 1920, Wald Collection, box 12, roll 10. Minutes of the Executive Committee Meeting of NOPHN, September 10, 1921, NOPHN Collection, roll 11.

108   Minutes of the Executive Committee Meeting of NOPHN, May 25–26, 1920, NOPHN Collection, roll 11; and Edna Foley to C.-E. A. Winslow, December 23, 1920.

109   "Editorial," *PHN* 12 (July 1920): 551–553.

110   "Memorandum," NOPHN Collection, June 14, 1920, CF-n21; and E. R. Embree to E. P. Crandall, June 18, 1920, NOPHN 1920 file; History 900–902, "Source Material," vol. 8, RF Archives, pp. 2085–2086. See also note 120.

111 Plans for their membership campaign were lagging behind schedule, and after what Foley called those "very awful sessions," they finally decided to go public. Edna Foley to C.-E. A. Winslow, December 23, 1920.

112 Sustaining (lay) members were chosen as the targets of this campaign because it was felt that little more money could be gotten from nurses. Minutes of the Staff Conference, November 30, 1920, NOPHN Collection, roll 27. Lillian Wald to Edna Foley, November 19, 1920, Wald Collection, box 12, roll 10. Lent was appointed executive director of the campaign, but by December, she had resigned. Two years later, she too left public health nursing to open an antique shop in New York City. Minutes of Board of Directors, January 20, 1921, NOPHN Collection, roll 11; and "Mary E. Lent," 60–62.

113 Minutes of the Executive Committee, NOPHN, November 23, 1921, Wald Collection, NOPHN folder, roll 31.

114 Edna Foley to Lillian Wald, May 9, 1921, Wald Collection, box 12, roll 10. Apparently, by December 1920, things seemed better. Bolton and Alexander White, Chairman of the Committee on Ways and Means, had, according to Foley, "been most generous." Foley to Wald, December 29, 1920. After her resignation, Foley evinced no further interest in NOPHN. Tucker discusses Foley's attitude after her visit to Chicago in Minutes of Staff Meeting, NOPHN, June 6, 1929, NOPHN Collection, roll 14.

115 Elizabeth Fox, "The Report of the Board of Directors," *PHN* 14 (September 1922): 452–455.

116 Ibid. Elizabeth Fox, "How Can We Finance Our Organization for Public Health Nursing?," *PHN* 13 (October 1921): 549–552; and Elizabeth Fox, "A Message to Our Members," *PHN* 13 (July 1921): 336–338.

117 Fox, "Report of the Board of Directors," 453.

118 Bolton "generously offered to contribute $20,000." Minutes of the Executive Committee, NOPHN, July 5, 1921, Wald Collection, roll 31; and Fox, "Message," 36–37.

119 Fox, "How?," 549–552.

120 Unfortunately, the NOPHN only had twelve contributors of such a generous nature. Fox, "How?," 551–552. In 1921, one-fifth of the budget came from nurse members, one-eighth from sustaining members, more than one-third from large contributors, and one-third from the American Red Cross, community chests, and foundations. The latter source of income was eliminated in 1922, and the number of large contributors significantly declined. Fox, "Report," 453. The Rockefeller Foundation was approached again in June of 1922. Vincent's reaction vas that the "so-called emergency" that the foundation had tried to eliminate with its first appropriation had apparently become a permanent problem and was not given serious consideration. G. G. Vincent interview with Anne Stevens, June 15, 1920, in "Report on the NOPHN," RF Archives, 1921, 22.75-n21. See also "Nonprofessional Membership in a Professional Organization," *PHN* 13 (August 1921): 383–384; and "Friends of Public Health Nursing," *PHN* 13 (January 1921): 9–15.

121 Minutes of the Board of Directors Meeting, December 10, 1920; and November 23, 1921, NOPHN Collection, roll 11; and Edna Foley to Lillian Wald, December 24, 1920.

122 Fox, "How?"; and Minutes of the Board of Directors Meeting, December 10, 1920, NOPHN Collection, roll 11.

123 Several other plans were considered between 1922 and 1924. One was a proposal of Mr. Clarence Burnet, who had been for nineteen years a financial secretary to

"organizations of national scope" and had acquired a list of 250,000 names—that is, a "virgin list." He promised, for a cost of 30 percent of money raised, to secure two hundred new members a day for the NOPHN. In the end, the board of directors voted to move more slowly and to use a "personal cultivation plan." Minutes of Board of Directors, January 17–18, 1923, NOPHN Collection, roll 11.

124 Minutes of the Staff Meeting, July 15, 1924b, NOPHN Collection, roll 14; and Elizabeth Fox, "The National Organization for Public Health Nursing Retrenches," *PHN* 16 (September 1924): 443–444. Both the ANA and the NOPHN appointed committees on self-analysis. On January 12, 1925, they voted that the time for a federation of the three nursing organizations had not yet arrived. Nursing still needed a purely professional organization, and public health nursing needed an organization that included lay memberships. Minutes of the Board of Directors Meeting, January 13–15, 1925, NOPHN Collection, roll 14.

125 Fox, "The NOPHN Retrenches," Minutes of the Staff Meeting, July 15, 1924, NOPHN Collection, roll 14; and Gardner, "What Are Voluntary Organizations to Do?," 458.

126 "Editorial," *PHN* 17 (November 1925): 598.

127 Minutes of the Executive Committee, October 8, 1925, NOPHN Collection, roll 11.

128 Minutes of Staff Meeting, March 24, 1926, NOPHN Collection, roll 14.

129 The conference included representatives from the New York, Brooklyn, Philadelphia, Pittsburgh, St. Louis, Detroit, Cleveland, Providence, New Haven, and Boston VNAs. Its underlying purpose was to get their response to the proposed percentage plan. "To Be or Not to Be," Minutes of the Meeting, December 18, 1925, NOPHN Collection, roll 25; and Theresa Kraker, "Activities of the NOPHN," *PHN* 18 (January 1926): 42–43.

130 Minutes of Staff Meeting, March 24, 1926, NOPHN Collection, roll 14; Mary Gardner, "Report of Six Months Study of the NOPHN," *PHN* 18 (July 1926): 374–386; "Editorial," *PHN* 18 (August 1926): 425; and "Future Plans for NOPHN," *Trained Nurse and Hospital Review* 18 (December 1926): 665–666.

131 Gardner, "Report of the Six Month Study," 374–386. The same recommendations were made again in April 1929 by the Committee of Programs and Policies, composed of Gardner, Sophie Nelson, and Patterson. Minutes of the Subcommittee to Consider Programs and Policies, April 20, 1929, NOPHN Collection, roll 11. As with the first Gardner Report, the executive committee again found these ideas so "stimulating and interesting" that they were published in an editorial in the *PHN*. "Future Service to Our Members," *PHN* 21 (June 1929): 283–284.

132 By 1930, only 29 percent of public health nurses belonged to the NOPHN. "The NOPHN," November 11, 1930, NOPHN Collection, roll 28; Anne Hanson, "Partial Report of the President," *PHN* 20 (July 1928): 340; Mary Beard, "A Nurse Looks at the Future," *PHN* 21 (May 1929): 257–259; Fox, "Past Challenges the Future," 275–278; and Elizabeth Fox, "How Shall We Use Our Opportunities?," *PHN* 18 (August 1926): 426–429.

133 Anne Hansen, "Local Responsibility for Support of National Health Agencies," *PHN* 19 (June 1929): 320–322. At the 1926 convention, the members voted to raise membership fees and charge for the *PHN*. The magazine would be $2.00 for members and $3.00 for nonmembers. Jane Allen, "Activities of the NOPHN," *PHN* 18 (September 1926): 513; "Financial Statement for 1927," *PHN* 20 (March 1928): 146; and Tucker, "Report of the General Director," 340–350.

134 "Board Member Forum," *PHN* 19 (May 1927): 245–246; Anne Hansen, "Convention Reports," *PHN* 20 (July 1928): 340–349; and "1927–1928" *PHN* 20 (January 1928): 2.

135 "Other Institutes," *PHN* 19 (May 1927): 247; and "One Day Institutes-Boston," *PHN* 20 (January 1928): 38–39. The papers given at the New Haven Institute can be found in the *PHN* 19 (June 1927): 293–333. Discussion related to Bolton's brother's gift can be found in Minutes of Staff Meeting, June 5, 1929, NOPHN Collection, roll 14. Although the executive committee was uncertain if the membership itself would find it acceptable, they hoped that eventually the NOPHN would have a lay president. This, they believed, would "greatly clarify . . . the whole question of the function of the NOPHN." Minutes of the Executive Committee, September 20–21, 1929; and January 16, 1930, NOPHN Collection, roll 11.

136 Minutes of Staff Meeting, June 5, 1929; and June 13, 1929, NOPHN Collection, roll 14.

137 "Meeting of the Largest VNA," December 18, 1925, NOPHN Collection, roll 25.

138 Wald realized the cutting down was difficult, but now that the clipping was done, she hoped the association would have a steadier and more healthful growth. July 13, 1922, Wald Collection, box 12, roll 10.

139 "Editorial," *PHN* 17 (November 1925): 545–548.

140 Crandall first worked for the New York Association for the Improvement of the Conditions of the Poor and from 1922 to 1926 for the American Child Hygiene Association. See also note 107. For Beard, see notes 24 and 107; for Lent, note 112. Even though Foley returned to Chicago to run their VNA, after her resignation from the NOPHN, she would have nothing further to do with it. See note 114. After two years of war work in France, LaMotte spent nearly a year in China. Her next book was *Peking Dust*. "Ellen Lamotte, Author, Was 87; Campaigner in 20s against Opium Traffic Is Dead—Cited by China, Japan," *New York Times*, March 4, 1961, 23. Frankel died in 1931. "Lee Frankel," *PHN* 23 (September 1931): 401.

141 Fitzpatrick, *National Organization*, 166–201.

142 Mary Gardner, *Public Health Nursing*, 3rd ed. (New York: Macmillan, 1936), 223.

143 Tattershall, "Census of Public Health Nursing," 266, 253.

144 See chapter 3. The attitude of NOPHN leadership was, not surprisingly, similar to that expressed at the turn of the century toward the ignorance of uninformed lady managers who threatened to drag down the standards of visiting nursing. "Editorial," *PHN* 16 (February 1924): 57; and Dorothy Deming, "Milestones of the Past Fifteen Years in Public Health Nursing," *AJPH* 29 (February 1939): 128–134.

145 See, for example, Henry Vaughan, "The Relation of the Public Health Nurse to the Practicing Physician: The Viewpoint of the Health Officer," *AJPH* 14 (February 1924): 114–118; and Ira Wiles, "The Relationship of the Public Health Nurse to the Practicing Physician: The Viewpoint of the Physician," *AJPH* 14 (February 1924): 106–111.

146 Wiles, "Relationship of the Public Health Nurse"; and J. G. Crownhart, "As Others See Us: The Public Health Nurse from the Standpoint of the Physicians," *PHN* 21 (July 1929): 343–345.

147 "Fixed Policies to Meet 'Fixed' Politics," *PHN* 18 (November 1926): 587–588; Mrs. Churchill Humphrey, "Point of View of the Contributing Citizen," *PHN* 18 (January 1926): 8–11; Elizabeth Fox, "Official County Health Work as It Affects Public Health Nursing," *PHN* 19 (December 1927): 594–598; Elizabeth Fox, "Meeting of the Provisional Public Health Nursing Section of APHA," *PHN* 15 (December 1923): 623–624; and Alta Dines, "The Relationship of Public Health Nurse to the Practicing Physicians: The Viewpoint of the Nurse," *PHN* 16 (March 1924): 111–114.

148 Fox, "Official County Health Work."

149 Ibid. Fox's audience was the joint membership of the health officers and public health nursing sections of the American Public Health Association (APHA).
Although they expressed them less extremely, other leading visiting nurses shared
these concerns. See, for example, Gardner, *Public Health Nursing*, 222–236,
452–459.
150 "Report of the Committee." Interestingly, Winslow was the chair of the committee, and Margaret Burkhardt, a visiting nurse, conducted the nursing part of the
survey. The MLI financed the study, which examined the current health practices
of eighty-three large municipal health departments in hopes of developing standards for practice. A supplement to the original schedule was sent to VNAs in
eighty-three cities so that comparison could be made between nursing staff of the
voluntary and official organizations. "Public Health Nursing: Abstract of Chapter
Forthcoming Report of the Committee on Municipal Health Practice," *AJPH* 12
(November 1922): 941–942; and Margaret Stack, "A Brief Report of Requirements
for Public Health Nurses in 83 Cities," *AJPH* 14 (January 1924): 22–24. The second
major study was American Child Health Association (ACHA), *A Health Survey of
86 Cities* (New York: ACHA, 1923). This study was conducted in 1923 and examined smaller cities. The last study was Ira Hiscock, "The Organization and Budget
of a Health Department in a City of 20,000 Population," *AJPH* 14 (March 1924):
203–208.
151 Stack, "Brief Report."
152 *Report of the Committee*; 19–20, 7; and ACHA, *Health Survey*, viii, 52–59.
153 "Editorial," *PHN* 16 (February 1924): 57.
154 Elizabeth Fox, "Public Health Nursing Section of the APHA," *PHN* 15 (January
1923): 623–624. In 1924, the executive committee voted that its major project for
the next year would be to study the organization and administration of nursing
services in state, county, and municipal health departments. Minutes of the Executive Committee, October 10–12, 1924, NOPHN Collection, roll 14. By 1927, this
remained a major concern of the NOPHN. Mary Beard's Diary, conversation with
Jane Allen (assistant director of NOPHN), July 27, 1927, RF Archives, RG 12.1.
Ella McNeil, "A History of the Public Health Nursing Section, 1922–1972" (APHA
1972), Boston University Archives, n97, box 1, folder 1, pp. 1–5. The idea of a
nursing section was mentioned as early as 1918, but it was not until 1920 that the
governing board took it under consideration.
155 C.-E. A. Winslow to Elizabeth Fox, December 23, 1921, Winslow Collection, 11:264.
156 Fox presented these views to the executive board of the APHA in a letter read by
Winslow. Minutes of the Executive Board of APHA, December 22, 1921, Boston
University Archives, n97, box 1, folder 1.
157 Ibid.
158 Elizabeth Fox, "A Section in Public Health Nursing," *PHN* 14 (September 1922):
441–442; McNeil, "Public Health Nursing Section"; and Margaret Stack, "Provisional Section Made Permanent," *PHN* 15 (December 1923): 608.
159 That NOPHN exercised some influence within the nursing section is confirmed
by the active participation of the NOPHN officers as well as by the nature of the
topics discussed during its early meetings. Early topics included amalgamation of
public and voluntary organizations, physician to public health nursing relationships, importance of follow-up in the home, generalized versus specialized services in agencies, and standardization of qualifications. McNeil, "Public Health
Nursing Section"; Alta Dines, "The Public Health Nurse at the Annual Meeting of

the APHA," *PHN* 17 (December 1925): 622; and Deming, "Milestones." The nursing section's growth was slow but steady, increasing from 126 in 1924 to 275 in
1930 and 537 by 1936. McNeil, "Public Health Nursing Section." That the APHA
rapidly incorporated the views and standards of the NOPHN is readily apparent
in all major studies and reports during this period. For an overview, see "Nursing
in Relation to the Three Plans Submitted for Municipal Health Practice," *PHN* 19
(March and April 1927): 130–134, 174–176. These three plans were as follows:
"Report of the Committee on Municipal Health Department Practices"; Hiscock,
"Organization and Budget"; and C.-E. A. Winslow and H. Harris, "An Ideal Health
Department for a City of 100,000 Population," *AJPH* 12 (November 1922): 891–905.
Emerson had also become very supportive of their views; see, for example, his
foreword in East Harlem Nursing and Health Service, *Comparative Study*; and
his articles, "The Visiting Nurse a County Service," *PHN* 15 (July 1923): 345–353;
and "Public Health Nursing—Indispensable and Economical for Everyone If Organized," *PHN* 22 (August 1930): 410–415. Probably the first joint committee was
appointed to establish qualifications for public health nursing positions. Its first
report can be found in Mabelle Welch, "Standardizing Qualifications for Public
Health Nurse Nursing Positions," *PHN* 17 (June 1923): 297–299. For its activities,
see Minutes of the Executive Committee, NOPHN, April 8, 1924; and October 10–
12, 1924, NOPHN Collection, roll 11. A second joint committee was appointed
in 1926 to study and report on the feasibility of advisory committees for official
public health nursing. See Fox, "Official County Health Work." Another was the
Committee on Administrative Practices. Interestingly, both organizations had such
a committee, but care was taken to make sure the nursing personnel were identi-
cal. Sophie Nelson, "Report of the Committee on Field Studies and Administrative
Practices," *PHN* 22 (July 1930): 350. Finally, there was also a joint committee to
study nursing services in the state departments of health.

160 This idea was studied and supported by the APHA Committee to Study Lay Committee Advisory Committees to Official Public Health Nursing Services in 1927 and
1930. See Fox, "Official County Health Work"; and Gardner, *Public Health Nursing*,
227–233.

161 W. F. Walker, "Analysis of Plans," *PHN* 19 (March 1927): 131. Not surprisingly,
the NOPHN was still expressing concern about the difficulty of specially trained
public health nurses fitting harmoniously into a health unit with a public health
officer who had had less preparation for his work than she had had for hers. "Conversation between Mary Beard and Jane Allen, General Director of the NOPHN,
July 27, 1927," Plans of M. Beard, RF, RG 12.1. By 1929, only 20 percent of America's rural population had access to a public health service under the direction of
a full-time health officer and only four hundred counties, out of approximately
2,160 rural counties in thirty-five states, had a full-time county health service.
Joseph Mountain, "County Health Organizations," *PHN* 21 (April 1929): 174–179;
and Minutes of the Executive Committee, NOPHN, October 7–8, 1927, NOPHN
Collection, roll 11.

162 NOPHN, *Survey of Public Health Nursing*, 1–10.

163 Ibid.; and Louise Tattershall, *Public Health Nursing in the United States. January 15, 1931* (New York: NOPHN, 1931). This survey was much more quantitative
than past NOPHN studies. Their sample represented a cross section of the country
and included twenty-eight communities, fifty-seven agencies, and the work of 960
public health nurses.

164 NOPHN, *Survey of Public Health Nursing*, 2.

165 Mabelle Welch, "What Is Public Health Nursing?," *AJN* 36 (May 1936): 452–456. This question is still being asked. See, for example, Carolyn Williams, "Community Health Nursing—What Is It?," *Nursing Outlook* 25 (April 1977): 250–254.

166 NOPHN, *Survey of Public Health Nursing*, 1–10.

167 Ibid., vii–viii.

168 Pearl McIver, "Some Findings of the NOPHN Survey of Public Health Nursing of Significance to State Health Administrators," *Public Health Reports* 49 (September 1934): 1081–1090.

169 NOPHN, *Survey of Public Health Nursing*, 14, 23, 31, 189.

170 Ibid., 14, 47, 52–53, 146.

171 Ibid., 23, 189.

172 Ibid., 31, 47, 53, 122–123, 155.

173 Ibid., 24, 30, 133, 145.

174 Ibid., 28–40; and McIver, "Some Findings," 1086–1087.

175 McIver, "Some Findings." The other criteria for performance were approach, technique, and adequacy of care. For all agencies and for all public health nursing services, the nurses' approach received the highest rating, while teaching was rated the lowest. While 74 percent of health departments, 96 percent of boards of education, and 87 percent of PHNAs required four years of high school for employment, 68 percent of health departments, 58 percent of boards of education, and 80 percent of PHNAs did not require any previous training or experience in public health nursing for employment. Louise Tattershall, "Pertinent Facts Relative to Salaries of Public Health Nurses," *PHN* 21 (November 1929): 605. In 1928 to 1929, only 275 nurses graduated from the eleven remaining postgraduate public health nursing certificate courses. "Students Registered in Accredited Courses," *PHN* 22 (January 1930): 40.

176 Tattershall, "Census of Public Health Nursing," 1–8.

177 Ibid.

Conclusion

1 The quotation by Winslow is from C.-E. A. Winslow, "Public Health Nursing," quoted by Allen Albert, "Nursing as a Social Influence," *AJN* 36(May 1936): 490.

2 Winslow "New Profession," 4, 128.

Suggested Readings

Compiled by Sandra Lewenson

Journal Articles

Abrams, Sarah. "From Function to Competency in Public Health Nursing." *Public Health Nursing* 21, no. 5 (October 2004): 507–510.

Apple, Rima. "School Health Is Community Health: School Nursing in the Early 20th Century in the United States." *History of Education Review* 46, no. 2 (2017): 136–149.

Apple, Rima D. "'Women's Mission among Women': Unacknowledged Origins of Public Health Nursing." *Nursing History Review* 26 (2018): 55–67.

Apple, Rima D., Ciara Breathnach, and Janet Greenless. "Evolving as Necessity Dictates: Home and Public Health in the 19th and 20th Centuries." *Nursing History Review* 26 (2018): 48–54.

Brown, Theodore M., and Elizabeth Fee. "Social Movements in Health." *Annual Review of Public Health* 35, no. 1 (2014): 385–398.

Buhler-Wilkerson, Karen. "Public Health Then and Now: Bringing Care to the People: Lillian Wald's Legacy to Public Health Nursing." *American Journal of Public Health* 83, no. 12 (December 1993): 1778–1782.

Connolly, Cynthia. "Nurses: The Early Twentieth Century Tuberculosis Preventorium Movement's 'Connecting Link.'" *Nursing History Review* 10 (2002): 127–157.

Connolly, Cynthia A., and Janet Golden. "'Save 100,000 Babies': The 1918 Children's Year and Its Legacy." *American Journal of Public Health* 108, no. 7 (2018): 902–907.

D'Antonio, Patricia. "Cultivating Constituencies: The Story of the East Harlem Nursing and Health Service, 1928–1941." *American Journal of Public Health* 103, no. 6 (2013): 988–996.

D'Antonio, Patricia. "Lessons Learned: Nursing and Health Demonstration Projects in New York City, 1920–1935." *Policy, Politics, and Nursing Practice* 14, nos. 3–4 (2014): 133–141. https://doi.org/10.1177/1527154413520389.

D'Antonio, Patricia, Cynthia Connolly, Barbra Mann Wall, and Julie Fairman. "Histories of Nursing: The Power and the Possibilities." *Nursing Outlook* 58 (2010): 207–213.

Flynn, Karen. "'Hotel Refuses Negro Nurse': Gloria Clarke Baylis and the Queen Elizabeth Hotel." *Canadian Bulletin of Medical History = Bulletin Canadien d'histoire de La Medecine* 35, no. 2 (2018): 278–308.

Frenk, Julio. "The Empowering Legacy of Academic Public Health." *Public Health Reports (1974–)* 131, no. 6 (2016): 851–854.

Gamble, Vanessa. "'Outstanding Services to Negro Health': Dr. Dorothy Boulding Ferebee and Dr. Virginia M. Alexander and Black Women Physicians' Public Health Activism." *American Journal of Public Health* 106 (2016): 1397–1404.

Gamble, Vanessa Northington. "'No Struggle, No Fight, No Court Battle': The 1948 Desegregation of the University of Arkansas School of Medicine." *Journal of the History of Medicine and Allied Sciences* 68 (2013): 377–415.

Gamble, Vanessa Northington. "'There Wasn't a Lot of Comforts in Those Days': African Americans, Public Health, and the 1918 Influenza Epidemic." *Public Health Reports* 125, no. 3 (2010): 114–125.

Green, Elna C. "Gendering the City, Gendering the Welfare State: The Nurses' Settlement of Richmond, 1900–1930." *Virginia Magazine of History and Biography* 113, no. 3 (2005): 276–311.

Gunn, Jennifer L. "Meeting Rural Health Needs: Interprofessional Practice or Public Health?" *Nursing History Review* 24 (2016): 90–97.

Hancock, Christina L. "Healthy Vocations: Field Nursing and the Religious Overtones of Public Health." *Journal of Women's History* 23, no. 3 (2011): 113–137.

Hawkins, Joellen, and John Charles Watson. "Public Health Nursing Pioneer: Jane Elizabeth Hitchcock 1863–1939." *Public Health Nursing* 20, no. 3 (June 2003): 167–176.

Hoffman, Steven. J. "Progressive Public Health Administration in the Jim Crow South: A Case Study of Richmond, Virginia, 1907–1920." *Journal of Social History* 35, no. 1 (September 2001): 175–194.

Jones, Marian Moser, and Matilda Saines. "The Eighteen of 1918–1919: Black Nurses and the Great Flu Pandemic in the United States." *American Journal of Public Health* 109 (June 2019): 877–884.

Kazanjian, Powel. "UNAIDS 90-90-90 Campaign to End the AIDS Epidemic in Historic Perspective." *Milbank Quarterly* 95, no. 2 (June 2017): 408–439.

Keeling, Arlene W. "Historical Perspectives on an Expanded Role for Nursing." *OJIN: The Online Journal of Issues in Nursing* 20, no. 2 (May 2015).

Kub, Joan, Pamela A. Kulbok, and Doris Glick. "Cornerstone Documents, Milestones, and Policies: Shaping the Direction of Public Health Nursing 1890–1950." *OJIN: The Online Journal of Issues in Nursing* 20, no. 2 (May 2015). https://doi.org/doi:10.3912/OJIN.Vol20No02Man03.

Kulbok, Pamela A., and Doris F Glick. "'Something Must Be Done!' Public Health Nursing Education in the United States from 1900 to 1950." *Family & Community Health: The Journal of Health Promotion & Maintenance* 37, no. 3 (September 2014): 170–178.

Kulbok, Pamela A., Joan Kub, and Doris Glick. "Cornerstone Documents, Milestones, and Policies: Shaping the Direction of Public Health Nursing 1950–2015." *Online Journal of Issues in Nursing* 22, no. 2 (May 2017): 4–4.1p.

Lewenson, Sandra. "Hidden and Forgotten: Being Black in the American Red Cross Town and Country Nursing Service, 1912–1948." *Nursing History Review* 27 (2019): 15–28.

Pittman, Patricia. "Rising to the Challenge: Re-embracing the Wald Model of Nursing." *American Journal of Nursing* 119, no. 7 (2019): 46–52.

Reverby, Susan M. "Ethical Failures and History Lessons: The U.S. Public Health Service Research Studies in Tuskegee and Guatemala M. Reverby, PhD." *Public Health Reviews* 34, no. 1 (2012): 1–18.

Rogers, Naomi. "Race and the Politics of Polio Springs, Tuskegee, and the March of Dimes." *American Journal of Public Health* 97, no. 5 (May 2007): 784–795.

Sano, Yulonda Eadie. "'Protect the Mother and Baby': Mississippi Lay Midwives and Public Health." *Agricultural History* 93, no. 3 (2019): 393–411.

Smith, Kylie M. "Different Places, Different Ideas: Reimagining Practice in American Psychiatric Nursing after World War I." *Nursing History Review* 26 (2018): 17–47.

Tuchman, Arleen Marcia. "Diabetes and Race: A Historical Perspective." *American Journal of Public Health* 101, no. 1 (2011): 24–33.

Weisz, George. "Epidemiology and Health Care Reform." *American Journal of Public Health* 101, no. 3 (March 2011): 438–447.

Wood, Pamela. "Historical Imagination and Issues in Rural and Remote Area Nursing." *Australian Journal of Advanced Nursing* 27, no. 4 (June 2010): 54–61.

Editorials

D'Antonio, Patricia. "The Great Flu and After: Why the Nurses?" *American Journal of Public Health* 109, no. 6 (June 2019): 832–833.

Swider, Susan M., Pamela F. Levin, and Pamela A. Kulbok. "Creating the Future of Public Health Nursing: A Call to Action." *Public Health Nursing* 32, no. 2 (2015): 91–93.

Discussion Papers

DeSalvo, Karen B., Y. Claire Wang, Andrea Harris, John Auerbach, Denise Koo, and Patrick O'Carroll. "Public Health 3.0: A Call to Action for Public Health to Meet the Challenges of the 21st Century." Discussion paper. Washington, D.C.: The National Academy of Medicine, 2017.

Books

Buhler-Wilkerson, Karen. *No Place like Home: A History of Nursing and Home Care in the United States.* Baltimore, Md.: John Hopkins University Press, 2001.

Chandler, Dana R., and Linda Kenny Miller. *To Raise Up the Man Farthest Down: Tuskegee University's Advancements in Human Health, 1881–1987.* Tuscaloosa: University of Alabama Press, 2018.

Cockerham, Ann, and Arlene Keeling. *Rooted in the Mountains, Reaching to the World: Stories of Nursing and Midwifery at Kentucky's Frontier School, 1939–1989.* Louisville, Ky.: Butler Books, 2012.

Connolly, Cynthia. *Saving Sickly Children: The Tuberculosis Preventorium in American Life: 1909–1970.* New Brunswick, N.J.: Rutgers University Press, 2008.

D'Antonio, Patricia. *American Nursing: A History of Knowledge, Authority, and the Meaning of Work.* Baltimore, Md.: Johns Hopkins University Press, 2010.

D'Antonio, Patricia. *Nursing with a Message: Public Health Demonstration Projects in New York City.* New Brunswick, N.J.: Rutgers University Press, 2017.

Fairman, Julie. *Making Room in the Clinic: Nurse Practitioners and the Evolution of Modern Health Care.* New Brunswick, N.J.: Rutgers University Press, 2008.

Feld, Marjorie N. *Lillian Wald: A Biography.* Chapel Hill: University of North Carolina Press, 2008.

Gebbie, Kristine, Linda Rosenstock, Lyla Hernandez M., and the Institute of Medicine of the National Academies, eds. *Who Will Keep the Public Healthy? Educating Public Health Professionals for the Twenty-First Century.* Washington, D.C.: National Academies Press, 2001.

Keeling, Arlene W. *Nursing and the Privilege of Prescription, 1893–2000.* Columbus: Ohio State University Press, 2007.

Mann Wall, Barbra. *Into Africa: A Transnational History of Catholic Medical Missionaries and Social Change.* New Brunswick, N.J.: Rutgers University Press, 2015.

Reverby, Susan M. *Examining Tuskegee: The Infamous Syphilis Study and Its Legacy.* Chapel Hill: University of North Carolina Press; 2009.

Robert Wood Johnson Foundation. *Catalysts for Change: Harnessing the Power of Nurses to Build Population Health in the 21st Century.* Princeton, N.J.: Robert Wood Johnson Foundation, 2017.

Rogers, Naomi. *Polio Wars: Sister Kenny and the Golden Age of American Medicine.* New York: Oxford University Press, 2014.

Smith, Susan L. *Sick and Tired of Being Sick and Tired: Black Women's Health Activism in America, 1890–1950.* Studies in Health, Illness, and Caregiving. Philadelphia: University of Pennsylvania Press, 1995.

Thomas, Karen Kruse. *Health and Humanity: A History of the Johns Hopkins Bloomberg School of Public Health, 1935–1985.* Baltimore, Md.: Johns Hopkins University Press, 2016.

Book Chapters

Apple, Rima D. "'Community Healthcare': Struggles and Conflicts of an Emerging Public Health System in the United States, 1915–45." In *Histories of Nursing Practice*, edited by Gerard M. Fealy, Christine E. Hallett, and Susanne Malchau Dietz, 163–179. Manchester, England: Manchester University Press, 2015.

Carthon, J. Margo Brooks. "Minority Nurses in Diverse Communities: Mary Elizabeth Tyler and the Whittier Centre in Early 20th-Century Philadelphia." In *Nursing History for Contemporary Role Development*, 3–18. New York: Springer, 2017.

Flynn, Karen. "Nurses Politically Engaged: Lillie Johnson and Sickle Cell Activism." In *Nursing History for Contemporary Role Development*, edited by Sandra Lewenson, Annemarie McAllister, and Kylie Smith, 181–204. New York: Springer, 2017.

Gibson, Mary Eckenrode. "School Nursing: A Challenging Strategy in Rural Health Care in the United States." In *Nursing History for Contemporary Role Development*, edited by Sandra B. Lewenson, Annemarie McAllister, and Kylie Smith, 37–58. New York: Springer, 2017.

Lewenson, Sandra. "Town and Country Nursing: Community Participation and Nurse Recruitment." In *Nursing Rural America: Perspectives from the Early 20th Century*, edited by John C. Kirchgessner and Arlene W. Keeling, 1–19. New York: Springer, 2015.

Smith, Kylie M., and Geertje Boschma. "Toward Community-Based Practice: The Changing Role of the Registered Nurse in Psychiatry and Mental Health." In *Nursing History for Contemporary Role Development*, edited by Sandra B. Lewenson, Annemarie McAllister, and Kylie Smith, 93–119. New York: Springer, 2017.

Index

ACHA. *See* American Child Health Association

acute care, x, xiii–xiv, xv

Adams, Phoebe, 3, 8

Aiken, Charlotte, 38

AJN. See American Journal of Nursing

Aldis, May, 126n14

amalgamation, 86–87, 163n57, 174–175n159

American Association for the Study of Prevention of Infant Mortality, 33

American Child Health Association (ACHA), 102

Americanization movement, 33, 43, 90

American Journal of Nursing (AJN), 166n71

American Medical Association, 92–93

American Nurses Association (ANA), 61, 88–89, 98, 104; NOPHN and, 53, 58, 72, 92, 97, 100, 166n71

American Public Health Association (APHA), 98, 102, 103–104, 105, 174n149, 174–175n159

American Society of Superintendents of Training Schools, 53

ANA. *See* American Nurses Association

APHA. *See* American Public Health Association

Baby Hygiene Association, Boston, Massachusetts, 25, 44, 130n51, 156n21

Baltimore, Maryland, 9, 24, 31, 119n33; Health Department, 26

Baltimore Charity Organization Society, Baltimore, Maryland, 9

Beale, Harriet Blaine, 147n67

Beard, Mary, 20, 24, 77, 128–129n42; background of, 127–128n39; at IDNA, 26–29, 79, 80–81, 130n58, 157n23; IDNA resignation attempts, 157–158n24; NOPHN and, 55, 66, 67, 72–73; at Rockefeller Foundation, 100, 157–158n24; World War I and, 64, 65, 67

bedside care, 70, 93; public health agencies and, 48, 69, 85, 87, 105, 160n43; rural nursing and, 63

Beer, A. E., 22–23

Biggs, Herman, 58, 65, 70, 77

Billings, John Shaw, 10

Blue, Rupert, 65

Boardman, Mabel, 60, 62, 93, 169nn92–93

boards of education, xviii, 34, 45, 101; employment of nurses, 48, 109

boards of health, xviii, 34, 45, 47, 101; employment of nurses, 48, 109; Red Cross affiliations, 61

Bolton, Chester, 71, 151n121

Bolton, Frances Payne, 51, 71–72, 96, 97, 120n43

Boston, Massachusetts, 22, 24, 25, 31, 79–80; district nursing in, 8; immigrants in, 123n64; patient demographics, 14; schools, 40–41; tuberculosis and, 43, 137–138n61

Boston Consumptive Hospital, Boston, Massachusetts, 137–138n61

Boston Dispensary, Boston, Massachusetts, 8, 25

Brainard, Annie, 20

Brewster, Mary, 10

Brown, Theodore, xiv

Bureau of Tuberculosis, Cleveland, Ohio, 42

Burns, Allen, 99

Cabot, Hugh, 24–25

Canada, 117–118n23

Cannon, Ida, 26

Carr, Ada, 11, 120–121n45

CHA. *See* Community Health Association, Boston

charitable organizations, 2, 7, 13

charity, 12, 27, 31, 55, 132–133n93; scientific, 9; stigma of, 56, 145n30, 146n57

Chicago, Illinois, 10, 24, 31, 70, 119n37; tuberculosis and, 43

About the Author

Karen Buhler-Wilkerson (1944–2010) was professor emerita, University of Pennsylvania School of Nursing, and director emerita of the Barbara Bates Center for the Study of the History of Nursing.

Available titles in the Critical Issues in Health and Medicine series:

Printed in the United States
By Bookmasters